Impl...
Mac...

GW01086934

System requirement:
- **Windows XP or above**
- **Power DVD player (Software)**
- **Windows media player version 10.0 or above**
- **Quick time player version 6.5 or above**

Accompanying DVD ROM is playable only in Computer and not in DVD player.

Kindly wait for few seconds for DVD to autorun. If it does not autorun then please follow the steps:
- Click on my computer
- Click the **drive labelled JAYPEE** and after opening the drive, kindly double click the file **Jaypee**

DVD Contents

1. Different procedures for implant treatment
2. Surgical procedure of implant placement
3. Two stage implant placement
4. Advance surgical implantology

Implantology Made Easy

TP Chaturvedi
BDS (Medalist), MDS (Lko), Fellow ICD, Fellow PFA

Incharge
Division of General Dentistry and Orthodontics
Faculty of Dental Sciences
Institute of Medical Sciences
Banaras Hindu University
Varanasi
(Uttar Pradesh) India

Ex-Chairman (HOD)
Department of Orthodontics and Dental Anatomy
Dr ZA Dental College, Aligarh Muslim University
Aligarh
(Uttar Pradesh) India

JAYPEE BROTHERS MEDICAL PUBLISHERS (P) LTD

New Delhi • Ahmedabad • Bengaluru • Chennai
Hyderabad • Kochi • Kolkata • Lucknow • Mumbai • Nagpur

Published by

Jitendar P Vij

Jaypee Brothers Medical Publishers (P) Ltd

B-3 EMCA House, 23/23B Ansari Road, Daryaganj, **New Delhi** 110 002
INDIA   Phones: +91-11-23272143, +91-11-23272703, +91-11-23282021
+91-11-23245672, Rel: +91-11-32558559   Fax: +91-11-23276490
+91-11-23245683, e-mail: jaypee@jaypeebrothers.com
Visit our website: www.jaypeebrothers.com

Branches

❑ 2/B, Akruti Society, Jodhpur Gam Road Satellite,
   Ahmedabad 380 015, Phones: +91-79-26926233, Rel: +91-79-32988717
   Fax: +91-79-26927094 e-mail: ahmedabad@jaypeebrothers.com
❑ 202 Batavia Chambers, 8 Kumara Krupa Road, Kumara Park East
   Bengaluru 560 001   Phones: +91-80-22285971, +91-80-22382956
   +91-80-22372664, Rel: +91-80-32714073   Fax: +91-80-22281761
   e-mail: bangalore@jaypeebrothers.com
❑ 282 IIIrd Floor, Khaleel Shirazi Estate, Fountain Plaza, Pantheon Road
   Chennai 600 008, Phones: +91-44-28193265, +91-44-28194897
   Rel: +91-44-32972089   Fax: +91-44-28193231
   e-mail:chennai@jaypeebrothers.com
❑ 4-2-1067/1-3, 1st Floor, Balaji Building, Ramkote, Cross Road
   Hyderabad 500 095   Phones: +91-40-66610020, +91-40-24758498
   Rel: +91-40-32940929   Fax:+91-40-24758499
   e-mail: hyderabad@jaypeebrothers.com
❑ Kuruvi Building, 1st Floor, Plot/Door No. 41/3098, B & B1, St. Vincent Road
   Kochi 682 018 Kerala   Phones: +91-484-4036109, +91-484-2395739
   Fax: +91-484-2395740   e-mail: kochi@jaypeebrothers.com
❑ 1-A Indian Mirror Street, Wellington Square
   Kolkata 700 013, Phones: +91-33-22651926, +91-33-22276404
   +91-33-22276415, Rel: +91-33-32901926   Fax: +91-33-22656075
   e-mail: kolkata@jaypeebrothers.com
❑ Lekhraj Market III, B-2, Sector-4, Faizabad Road, Indira Nagar
   Lucknow 226 016 Phones: +91-522-3040553, +91-522-3040554
   e-mail: lucknow@jaypeebrothers.com
❑ 106 Amit Industrial Estate, 61 Dr SS Rao Road, Near MGM Hospital, Parel
   Mumbai 400 012   Phones: +91-22-24124863, +91-22-24104532
   Rel: +91-22-32926896, Fax: +91-22-24160828
   e-mail: mumbai@jaypeebrothers.com
❑ "KAMALPUSHPA" 38, Reshimbag, Opp. Mohota Science College
   Umred Road, **Nagpur** 440 009 Phone: Rel: +91-712-3245220
   Fax: +91-712-2704275 e-mail: nagpur@jaypeebrothers.com

Implantology Made Easy

© 2008, Jaypee Brothers Medical Publishers

First Edition: **2008**

ISBN 81-8448-160-8

Typeset at   JPBMP typesetting unit
Printed at   Ajanta Offset & Packagings Ltd., New Delhi

Contributors

Dr Farhan Durrani
MDS (Periodontics)
Lecturer, Division of Periodontics
Faculty of Dental Sciences, IMS, BHU, Varanasi
(Certificate American Academy of Implant Dentistry)

Dr Geeta
MDS (Prosthodontics)
IMS, BHU, Varanasi

Dr AS Rana
MDS (Oral and Maxillofacial Surgery)
Subharati Dental College
Meerut

Professor BP Singh
Dean, Faculty of Dental Sciences,
IMS, BHU, Varanasi

Preface

There has been unprecedented enhancement and advancement in last few decades in implant dentistry. Scope of implantology is increasing by leaps and bound. The work of Branemark was tremendous, probably gives new vision for implant science and also gives good direction in various areas of implant success and research. Implant subject is not very well covered by Dental Council of India for undergraduate as well as postgraduate dental curriculum for dental students as a separate course and also every practitioner is not aware of it. It is essential to know as well as understand basic use and application of implants for every students and practitioners. The implant system currently available are diverse. There are at least many companies manufacturing different implant systems. Manufacturers have developed individualized designs for their implants, and they are continually altering marketing strategies to highlight the feature of each implant. They themselves describe from case selection to completion of implant placement and prosthetic treatment procedures.

Objective of present book is to give some basic information related to implants right from its inception to use in dentistry in proper way. I have tried to incorporate basic, relevant and important feature of implants applicable to every system of implant placement. I have tried to give one special chapter 'Literature Revisited' to give an insight into development that is taking place in implantology from early time. It is not only a complete book for those who are making implantology as their career but also quite useful for dental students and practitioners to understand implants in a proper way for their clinical use and day-to-day practice. Your suggestions and modifications for this book are always welcome.

TP Chaturvedi

Acknowledgements

Objective of present book is to introduce basic and expanding field of implant dentistry to dental practitioners and students. I would like to thank Dr Farhan Durrani, Lecturer in Division of Perio-dontics, Faculty of Dental Sciences, IMS, BHU, Varanasi and Professor BP Singh, Dean and Head Division of Prosthodontics, Faculty of Dental Sciences, IMS, BHU, Dr Geeta, MDS in Prostho-dontics for the co-operation and help provided by them in completing this book. My great respect for Professor Vakil Singh, Department of Metallurgical Engineering, IT, BHU who is in process of making of indigenous implant which is quite economical and well suited for Indian Population and quite successfully used in the Dental Department of BHU.

My deepest regards to my students and my friends specially from Dr ZA Dental College, AMU, Aligarh who has supported me in writing this book. I would like to thank IDA members of UP State for proper guidance and encouragement for completion of this book. I thank all my teachers and friends in KGMC Lucknow (now become KGDU) who supported and contributed me time-to-time. This work would not have been possible without the support of my parents, wife Renu and sons Hemang and Kushagra. *This work is completed because of the divine blessings of almighty God.*

Contents

CHAPTER
1

Introduction, History and Uses of Implants

INTRODUCTION

The goal of modern dentistry is to restore the patient to normal contour, function, comfort, esthetics, speech, and health, regardless of the atrophy, disease or injury of stomatognathic system. Teeth are integral part of the stomatognathic system. The primary function of teeth is to prepare food for swallowing as well as to initiate and facilitate digestion. Teeth are also necessary for the articulation of speech and proper looks.

Normal versus abnormal anatomy from tooth generates a compromised repaired structure both in function and form. A balance of force provides an anatomically steady-state when teeth are present. With loss of even one tooth element, however steady-state is broken and a variety of progressive changes takes place. Loss of tooth/teeth results in loss of structural balance, inefficient oral function and poor esthetics. Besides caries, periodontal disease and positional changes of remaining natural teeth, the edentulous state may lead to a feeling of inconvenience and sometimes severe handicapness. Hence, replacement of the lost tooth/teeth is essential to maintain the occlusal function and optimum oral health apart from its masticatory and esthetic needs. Also the feeling of inconvenience and handicapness can be avoided by replacement of teeth. Several methods are being used for replacement of missing tooth/teeth with natural or synthetic substitutes since centuries.

Conventional rehabilitation methods include tissue supported, tooth supported or dual supported removable dentures. Acrylic removable partial dentures are very common, as they are very economical. But removable partial dentures have certain drawbacks such as reduced masticatory efficiency and discomfort due to soft tissue support, difficulty in speech due to prosthesis size (palate and flanges), inconvenience and lack of confidence in patients due to less retentive prosthesis. The patients wearing partial dentures often exhibit greater mobility of abutment teeth, plaque retention, increased bleeding on probing, more incidences of caries and accelerated bone loss in the edentulous regions.

Another modality of restoration of missing teeth is fixed partial denture, which takes the support of adjacent teeth. Fixed partial dentures provide better masticatory efficiency, comfort and added confidence to patients. But, it needs the preparation of the adjacent healthy teeth. Further caries, sensitivity and periodontal disease of the abutments are seen in fixed partial denture patients in the long-term.

The latest modality of treatment of partial and completely edentulous patients is dental implants (Figs 1.1 and 1.2). Dental implants are made of

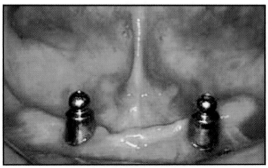

Fig. 1.1: Endosteal implant

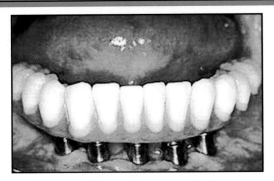

Fig. 1.2: Implant supported fixed prosthesis in lower arch

biocompatible materials and they are surgically inserted into the jawbone primarily as a prosthodontic foundation. The endosteal dental implants or root form implants are commonly used. Endosteal dental implants are similar to the natural tooth root and restoration of missing teeth does not need adjacent tooth support primarily. Also, implant stimulates the supporting bone and maintains its dimensions similar to that of healthy roots. Implant supported prosthesis does not require soft tissue support and improves oral comfort. Thus, implant supported prosthesis offers several advantages over the removable and fixed partial dentures.

HISTORY

'The first sub-periosteal implant was originally developed and placed in the United States by Gershokoff and Goldberg in 1949. Later on thousands of such implants have been placed. But, the advent of two-stage endosseous root form implants has affected those sub-periosteal cases that have more than 10 mm of residual vertical bone available in the symphyseal area of the mandible. Also the transmandibular implant may be an option for cases with less than 7 mm of the vertical symphyseal bone.

The endosseous implants may be root forms or blade forms. The root form implants are most often used for the restoration of partially or completely edentulous arches.

The ancient Chineese 4000 years ago, Egyptians 2000 years ago and Incas 1500 years ago knew to use the root form implants. The most recent history was in 1809, Maggiolo introduced the usage of gold in the shape of the tooth root. In 1887, Harris reported the usage of porcelain and in early 1900s. Lambotte fabricated implants of many materials and identified corrosion of these metals in the body tissues. In 1909, Greenfield gave latticed cage design, made of iridioplatinum. In 1938, Strock introduced surgical cobalt chromium molybdenum alloy for implantation. He designed a two-stage screw implant in 1946 that was implanted without a permucosal post. The first submerged implant placed by Strock was functioning even 50 years later.

The implant interface was described then as "ankylosis", which may be equated to the clinical term "rigid fixation".

In 1948, Formiggini, developed the first successful metal spiral screw implant and is regarded as the "Father of Modern Endosseous Implantology".

In 1960, titanium blade implant was introduced by Linkow. In 1987, Weiss stated the development of a functionally oriented, peri-implant connective tissue that dampen or absorb the forces of mastication, "the fibro-osseous integration". An initial clinical report gives the restoration of a maxillary lateral incisor with blade type implants in a case of narrow ridge of 1.2 mm width, with a clinical success of 12 years. Some examples of the blade forms are Biolox (fabricated from aluminum oxide) and Osteoplate-2000, Oraltronics.

The term "osseointegration" was first defined by Branemark. He did extensive experimental studies on the microscopic circulation of bone marrow healing which greatly influenced the implant concepts. One of the best known implant system used worldwide is the Branemark system. In 1965; 'Branemark implants' were placed in patients for the first time. They were of screw-type implants made of pure titanium, without any special surface modification.Unlike his predecessors, Branemark studied every aspect of implant design, including biological,mechanical,physiogical and functional phenomena relative to the success of the endosteal implant.

The intramobile cylinder (IMZ) has been used clinically since 1974, which has an elastic compensating component inserted between the implant and the prosthetic superstructure.

The elastic intramobile element acts as a periodontal ligament of a natural tooth providing shock absorption and also a force distribution. The IMZ system is made available with surface coatings (such as titanium plasma spray and apatite coating). In the same year (1974), the Tubingen implant was developed by Prof Schulte. The Frialit-Tubingen immediate implant is the first root-shaped implant system adapted to the socket, made of bio-ceramic with regularly spaced lacunae. The Frialit-2 implant system introduced later (1992) is a root analog stepped design in the form of stepped cylinders and stepped screws. The ITI Bonefit implant system was developed by the "International Team for Implantology' (ITI) and consists of three different basic types: hollow cylinder, hollow screw and solid screw, may be a single-stage or a two-stage system. The two stage system is placed transgingivally in contrast to other systems. In 1977, the Straumann Co. in collaboration with Dr Phillipe Ledermann, developed the TPS (Titanium Plasma Sprayed) screw type implant similar to the single stage ITI screw implant. This implant was mainly designed to use in the edentulous mandible. The Ha-Ti (Hand-Titanium) implant system clinically used since 1985 is a conical, step-screw, pure titanium implant with self tapping threads.

For centuries, people have attempted to replace missing teeth using implantation.

In this way there are over 100 different dental implant systems commercially available world wide for the restoration of partially or completely edentulous arches. 'To a beginner, restoration using the dental implants has become difficult as one has to choose the right implant system. Also it is important to know that the Council on Dental Materials, Instruments and Equipment (CDMIE) which is an arm of American Dental Association (ADA) has established an "acceptance program" to set standards for implant quality control.

SCOPE OF IMPLANT TREATMENT

Over the last decade, reconstruction with implants has changed considerably. Implants are basically used in prosthetic rehabilitation in edentulous, partially edentulous, and single tooth cases. Its applications in new areas such as maxillofacial prosthodontics, the anchoring of hearing aids and in orthodontic therapy are also considered nowadays. If the potential benefits of such uses are to be maximized, then it is essential that implant treatment be selected on logical basis and placed within the context of the full range of treatment modalities available in restorative dentistry. Today's implants practitioner considers a broad and complex set of interwoven factors before formulating an implant-treatment plan. The entire scope of treatment has progressed originally from the tooth replacement to surgically oriented implant reconstruction and more restorative approach for rehabilitation of stomatognathic system.

SUMMARY

The use of endosteal implants for dental rehabilitation of patients represents one of the most technologically advanced forms of dentistry available today. Endosteal implants are effective and appropriate for replacing single teeth, as well as for rehabilitating edentulous arches. Basic advantage of implants is to preserve the alveolar bone similar to the healthy tooth. Dental implants can stabilize maxillofacial prosthesis. With the help of all health care professionals involved in the care of these patients will increase success rates.

CHAPTER

2

Types of Implants

Dental implant treatment has been one of the most recent success stories of dentistry. The use of dental implants in the treatment of complete and partial edentulism has become an integral treatment modality in prosthetic dentistry. Dental implants are made of biocompatible (materials relatively inert) material and they are surgically inserted into the jawbone primarily as a prosthetic foundation. They may be endosteal implants, periosteal implants, transosteal implants according to their relationship to the bone.

The endosteal dental implants or root form implants are commonly used. Endosteal dental implants are similar to the natural tooth root and restoration of missing teeth primarily does not need adjacent tooth support. Also, implant stimulates the supporting bone and maintains its dimensions similar to that of healthy roots. Implant supported prosthesis does not require soft tissue support and improves oral comfort. Thus, implant supported prosthesis offers several advantages over the removable and fixed partial dentures.

IMPLANT CLASSIFICATION

Dental implants may be broadly classified in relationship to the bone and the biomaterials used. They may be endosteal, periosteal, transosteal in relationship to the bone.

Endosteal Implant

It is device that placed into the alveolar and/or basal bone of the mandible or maxilla transects only one cortical plate. The endosteal implants may be the root form or the blade form implants (Figs 2.1A and B). These implants are formed in different shapes, such as cylindrical cones or thin plates, and can be used in all areas of the mouth. One example of endosteal implant is blade implant consists of thin plates embedded into bone, they are used for narrow spaces such as posterior edentulous areas, their application in modern implantology is minimal.

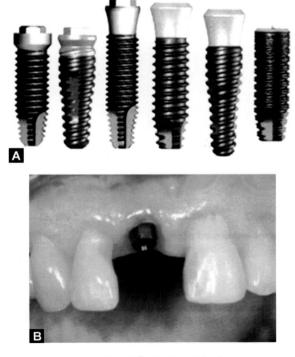

Figs 2.1A and B: Endosteal implants

The root form implants use a vertical column of bone similar to the root of natural tooth. The term "root form" is recognized by the American Academy of Implant Dentistry in 1988. The root forms offer the advantages such as usage in multiple intraoral locations, uniformly precise implant site preparation and the cost of failure similar to the tooth loss. They may be described based on the shape of the implant, the implant abutment interface, abutment connection and also the implant surface and coating.

Sub-periosteal Implants

It employs an implant substructure and superstructure. The custom cast frame is directly beneath the periosteum overlying the bony cortex. It can be used to restore partially dentate or completely edentulous jaws and is used when there inadequate bone for endosseous implants. Disadvantage of this implants are slow but predictable rejection of implants, difficult retrievability, and excessive bone loss associated with failure (Figs 2.2A to C).

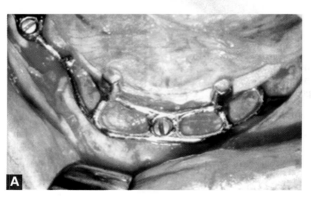

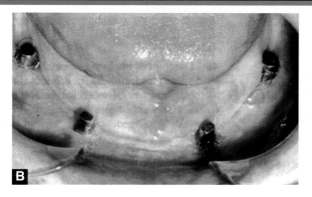

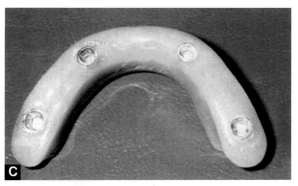

Figs 2.2A to C: (A) Sub-periosteal implant positioned beneath the periosteum (B) Superstructure for sub-periosteal implant allowing for attachment of prosthesis (C) Denture restoration for sub-periosteal implant

Transosteal Implants

It combines the both sub-periosteal and endosteal components. This type of implants penetrates both cortical plates and passes through the full thickness of the alveolar bone. This type of implants is

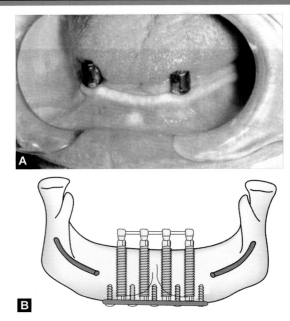

Figs 2.3A and B: (A) Transmucosal abutment for transosteal implant allowing for placement of denture restoration (B) Transosteal implant

restricted to anterior area of mandible and provides support for tissue born overdentures (Figs 2.3A, B and 2.4).

Epithelial Implant

This is inserted into the oral mucosa. It is no longer used.

IMPLANT MACRODESIGN

They may be of three primary types: cylinder root forms, screw root forms and combination forms (Fig. 2.5).

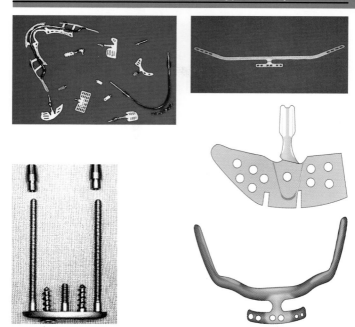

Fig. 2.4: Different types of transosseous pin smooth staple implant with top plate and accessories used for atrophic mandible

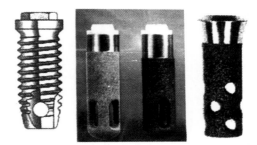

Fig. 2.5: Threaded screw, cylinder and hollow basket

Cylinder Root Forms

The primary stability of the cylindrically shaped implant is a function of the dimensional difference between the implant bed and the diameter of the inserted implant, as well as the micro-interlocking (surface roughness) of the implants. Some of the variations of the press-fit cylinders are straight cylinder (IMZ), cylinders with steps, screws (Frialit) and hollow basket cylinder (Straumann Co). Other press-fit forms are truncated cone-shaped design (Endopore system), finned taper design (Bicon implants) (Fig. 2.6).

The cylinder design implant system offers advantage of ease of placement even in difficult access locations and in the very soft type 4 bone. Most cylinder type implants are either smooth sided or bullet shaped and require a bioactive surface or a coating to increase the surface area for better retention in bone.

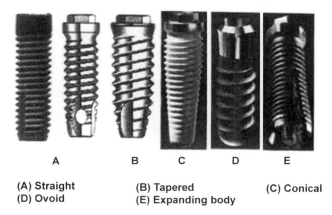

| A | B | C | D | E |

(A) Straight   (B) Tapered   (C) Conical
(D) Ovoid   (E) Expanding body

Fig. 2.6: Threaded screws

Screw Forms

The screw form implants are threaded into a bone site and have macroscopic retentive elements for initial bone fixation. The common thread shapes in implant designs are square, V-shaped and buttress threads. The V-threads result in tenfold increase in shear at the implant to bone interface compared with square (power) thread design. The buttress threads result in comparable shear as V-threads at the implant bone interface.

Some of the threaded screw variations are straight, tapered, conical, ovoid and expanding body. Some examples are Branemark screw, ITI Bonefit screw, Ledermann screw, TPS Screw, etc. The new screw designs include pan head screws with fewer threads and long shank for optimal elongation (Fig. 2.7).

Combination Root Forms

They possess macroscopic features of both cylinder and screw root forms. Some of the other features

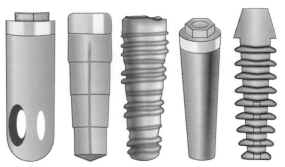

Fig. 2.7: Press-fit cylinders

are, the natural taper which closely approximates the natural root profile; vented taper; cupped recesses which act as a repository for bone shavings; domed apical end which reduces trauma and is desirable for sinus lift procedures and incremental cutting edge which lessen the torque and reduces friction.

THE IMPLANT ABUTMENT INTERFACE

The implant is connected to the abutment by coupling which is external about 2 mm superior to the coronal surface of the implant and internal about 5 mm internal to the coronal surface of the implant body. The external connection is either a standard hexagonal or octagonal with 0.7-l mm platform (Figs 2.8 and 2.9).

The internal connection may be a slip-fit or a friction fit. Slip-fit is a passive fit of the abutment

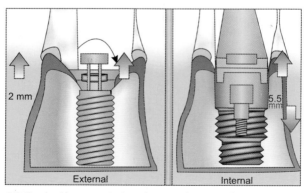

Fig. 2.8: Implant is connected to abutment by a coupling. External about 2 mm superior to the coronal surface of implant. Internal about 5 mm inferior to coronal surface to implant

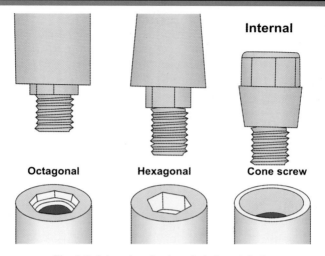

Octagonal   Hexagonal   Cone screw

Fig. 2.9: Internal and external abutment design

part to the implant, such as octagonal, hexagonal, cone screw with a non rotational feature, cylindrical hex and cam tube or cam tube or cam cylinder. The deep internal hexagon is reported to be the most preferred one. The friction fit provides a locking taper and have no gap between the mating components, thus preventing bacterial leakage.

The Abutment Connection

The abutment is the portion of the implant that supports and/or retains prosthesis or super-structures. The abutment may be in the form of an overdenture ball attachment, screw retention or cement retention. The abutment for screw retention have variations such as flat top, conical, ULCA plastic, ULLCA variations (Aurabase, Auraadapt.) and those for cement retention may be straight shoulderless, shoulder abutments [Ceraone, STA (3i)], etc. Some esthetic abutments, e.g. Cerabase (ceramic abutment with metal base), Ceradapt (ceramic direct connection abutment) are made of high quality ceramics.

DESIGN OF IMPLANTS

It should fulfill the following requirements:
- Easily placed with least trauma to bone
- Should have antirotational properties so that it does not come out
- Should distribute the loads evenly throughout the bone bed
- Should be restorable in such a way that it can be maintained by both patient as well as clinician for the health of soft and hard tissues
- Should be good enough to avoid fatigue fracture after long-term service in patient's mouth
- If needed, it should be retrievable with relative ease.

Implant Components

Although each implant system varies, the parts are basically consistent (Fig. 2.10).

1. *The first part is fixture (endosteal root form) or dental implant body:* It actually engages bone. Depending on the implant system, the fixture can have different surfaces—Threaded, grooved, perforated, plasma sprayed or coated. Each surface type is meant to serve a particular purpose, for example increased surface area enhances osseointegration ensures immediate and long-term bone anchorage.

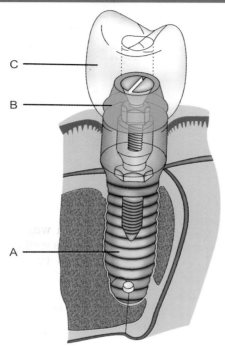

Fig. 2.10: Diagram of implant components (A) The implant fixture (endosteal root form) (B) Transmucosal abutment that serves as the attachment between fixture and the actual prosthesis (C) The actual prosthesis that can either be cemented, screwed or swaged

Implant may either be of a multipart design which is intended to be buried while osteointegration occurs, or a single part design, which will penetrate the mucosa from the time of placement (Figs 2.11A to D). Multipart designs incorporate various mechanical linkages to facilitate the joining of the different components and mechanical integrity of the joint. These usually

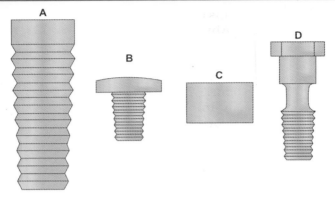

Figs 2.11A to D: Components used in dental implantology (A) A threaded tapered implant body (B) Cover screw, used to cover the top of the implant (C) Parallel-sided transmucosal abutment and (D) An abutments screw; this is used to secure the abutment to the implant body

include a hexagonal socket on one component to provide resistance to rotation, or a tapered joint to provide both this and seal. The joint is commonly held closed by a screw, although some manufactures employ fixation.

Cover screw (dental implant obturator): This is a placed at the time of first stage surgery, and removed when locating the abutments. Where the implant body is not internally threaded the description 'screw' is inappropriate. The term dental implant obturator is also used for cover screw.

2. *Implant abutment or transmucosal abutment:* Second component is the transmucosal abutment which provides the connection between the implant fixture and prosthesis that will be fabricated. Abutment actually connected to the

fixture by means of screw, it can also be cemented or swaged. Abutment can engage either an internal or external hexagon on the fixture that serves as an antirotation device, which is particularly important for single unit restorations. It can be cylindrical designs, shouldered designs. Since the bony anatomy places constraints on the location and orientation of a dental implant, sometimes angulated abutment is used.

It is typically a machined or custom-made component. These abutments may be made in a dense ceramic, CPTi or gold alloy. Advantage of machined abutment are that it is simple to use, requires minimal chairside and laboratory time and has a predictable precision fit and good retention. A customized abutment may be prepable, custom-made in the laboratory or computer-aided design/computer-aided-manufacture (CAD/CAM) designed (Figs 2.12A to F and 2.13A to E).

Healing abutment: This is temporary implant connecting part placed on the implant body to create a channel through the mucosa while the adjacent soft tissues heal.

Impression coping: This is also described as a dental implant impression cap and is used to transfer the position of the implant body or the abutment to the working cast.

Healing cap: Most manufacturers provide temporary polymeric covers for their abutments to prevent damage and fouling of the screw retainer when the patient has to be without the superstructure during its fabrication or repair.

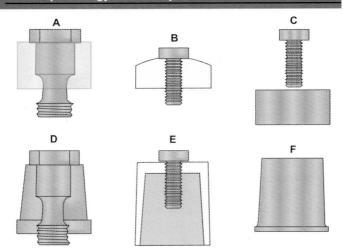

Figs 2.12A to F: Implant components. A standard abutment complete with screw (A) and the associated healing cap (B) and gold cylinder (C) when using tapered abutments (D) a special tapered healing cap (E) should be employed, while a pre-manufactured gold cylinder (F) is incorporated into the prosthesis to provide a precise and secure linkage with the underlying implant

3. Last part of an implant is the prosthesis attached to the abutment through the use of screws, cement, or precision attachments, such as those used for implant overdentures.

Implant to abutment connection and implant to final prosthesis connection:

• A final prosthesis may be connected to the implant in several ways;
  Screw retained direct to implant
  Screwed joints Screwed joint are functions by virtue of its components being held tightly

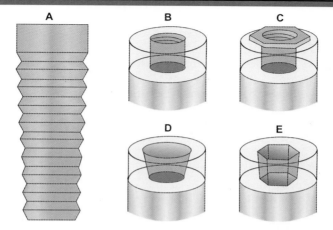

Figs 2.13A to E: Examples of the principles of some of the methods used manufacturers to link implant abutments of the implant itself

together by the tension in the screw. Some manufactures recommend routine checking of screw tightness after a short period of time.

Advantages

- Retrievability:
  - Easy to remove
  - Aids the checking of various connecting components, abutments and surrounding soft tissue
  - Conveniently remounted on a dental cast for analysis and modification in the laboratory.
- Control of gap:
  - It can be precise
  - Occlusal adjustments in laboratory will be more accurate

- No cement breakdown or extrusion from joint at time of placement.
- Predictable Failure:
  - Screwed joints can be designed to be weakest part of linkage and thus fail preferentially
  - This can protect other components from mechanical overload
  - No risk of excess cement in soft tissues
  - Decrease in clinical and laboratory time.

Disadvantages

- Mechanical failure—It can be problematical
- Access holes—It is necessary for screw placement which may penetrate the prosthesis at an aesthetically unfavorable site or compromise the occlusion
- Increased bulk of cingulum in anterior teeth
- Contamination—It can permit ingress of material and microorganisms from the mouth. Some screwed joints incorporate a tapered design, which provide a seal between the components, while others may include a synthetic rubber O-ring to reduce the risk of oral bacteria infecting deeper tissues
- Angulations problems—It may be very difficult to manage where long axis of crown diverges markedly from that implant body.

Cemented Joints

Advantages

- Simplicity—It requires clinical and laboratory techniques similar to conventional crown and bridgework
- Passivity—Accuracy of fits not as critical as with screw retention

- Angulation—It can be used where the projection of the long axis of the implant body would penetrate the labial or buccal aspect of restoration
- It improves esthetics in the absence of occlusal access holes.

Disadvantages
- Retrievability may be difficult
- Excess cement may be extruded into soft tissues
- Dimensions—Cementation needs to be controlled otherwise, occlusion of the final prosthesis may not be correct
- Increased cost of production.

SUMMARY

There is a long history and well documented data on the success of dental implants. The field of implant dentistry has seen many advances in the last two decades putting forth wide range of choices to the clinician. Therefore, the commercially available implant systems have to be considered based on the simplicity, ease in placement, clinical studies and follow-up data before using them in clinical practice. A broad classification is also essential to place all the acceptable implant-systems giving an insight to their principles, and concepts.

CHAPTER
3

Implant Osseointegration

For centuries, people have attempted to replace missing teeth using implantation. Implantation is defined as insertion of any object or material, such as an alloplastic substance or other tissue, either partially or completely, into the body for therapeutic, diagnostic, prosthetic, or experimental purposes. In 1952 Branemark developed a threaded implant design made of pure titanium that increased the popularity of implants to new levels. Branemark studied every aspect of implant design, including biological, mechanical, physiological and functional phenomenon relative to the success of the endosteal implant.

IMPLANT ATTACHMENT

Periodontal fibers, which attach a tooth to the bone, consist of highly differentiated fibrous tissue. These fibers are with numerous cells and nerve endings that allow for shock absorption, sensory function, bone formation, and tooth movements. Although this is most ideal form of attachment, there is no known implant material or system at present that can stimulate the growth of these fibers and mimic the function of a natural tooth.

Historically, implant attachment through low-differentiated fibrous tissue was widely accepted as a measure of a successful implant placement. However, it was later learned that this type of attachment is a manifestation of adverse reactions that later lead to implant failure. Such reactions include tissue rejection where an acute or chronic inflammatory response is accompanied by pain and eventual loss of the implant. Another manifestation is implant encapsulation by poorly differentiated fibers that have been called a "pseudo-periodontium."Clinical studies indicate that this type of attachment can eventually lead to an acute rejection or acute reaction, and progressive looseness will occur.

OSSEOINTEGRATION

Extensive work by Swedish orthopedic surgeon Branemark led to discovery that commercially pure titanium (CPTi), when placed in a suitably prepared site in the bone, could become fixed in place due to close bond between the two, a phenomenon that he later described as osseointegration(OI). This mode is described as the direct adaptation of bone to implants without any other intermediate interstitial tissue, and it is similar to a tooth ankylosis where no periodontal ligament exists. Integration occurs initially through osteoconduction wherein bone producing cells migrates along side of the implant surface through connective tissue scaffolding formed adjacent to implant surface. Following factors influence Implant osseointegration.

Implant Design

Implant design has great influence on the stability and subsequent function of the implant in bone. The main parameters are implant shape, implant length, and implant diameter as well as surface characteristics.

Root form implants such as screws and cylinders are the dominating implant designs today. Screw implants are considered to be superior to cylindrical ones in terms of initial stability and resistance to compression and tension stresses under loading.

Implant Length

Implant length varies from 6-20 mm, most common lengths are employed are between 8-15 mm. Within anatomical limitation, it is good practice to use the longest implant that can be safely placed, with, wherever possible bicortical stability.

Implant Diameters

The diameter of most implants falls within the range of 3.3-6 mm. Narrow diameter implants can be used in small spaces. Larger diameter implants may be used in, particular in posterior areas of the mouth and where there is poor quality bone.

Surface Characteristic

It has been suggested that the quality of osseo-integration is related to the physical and chemical nature of the surface of the implant. Increasing surface roughness increases the bone to implant contact area and in turn osseointegration.

The Host Site

Bone Factors

There are difference in the anatomy of the bone of the maxilla and the mandible. Higher ratio of compact to cancellous bone exists in the mandible. Bone density has been found to be an important factor in the initial stability and prevention of micromovement of the implant. Sectional tomograms and computed tomography scans provide an indication of medullary bone density. From a clinical point of view, the quality of bone can be assessed during surgery, based on subjective feel and by assessing cutting resistance during drilling, tapping and placement of the implant (Figs 3.1A to D). (Classification of Lekoholm and Zarb as well as Cawood and Howell) Bone volume does not itself influence osseointegration, but is an important determinant of implant placement. Where bone bulk is lacking then small implants may need to be used, with the consequent risk of mechanical overload and implant failure.

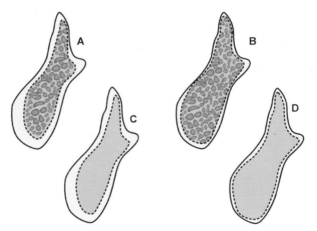

Figs 3.1A to D: A scheme for classifying patterns of bone in the edentulous jaw. (A) Thick cortex and plentiful cancellous bone (B) Thin cortex and plentiful cancellous bone (C) Dense cortex with minimal cancellous bone; and (D) Sparse cancellous bone and a thin cortex. All can provide effective support for a dental implant however, there is an increased risk of thermal trauma in types A and C, and problems are often encountered obtaining good primary fixation in types B and D

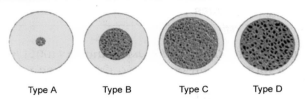

Type A   Type B   Type C   Type D

Figs 3.2A to D: Four types of bone ranging from homogenous compact bone to low density trabecular bone (Classification given by KJ Anusavice)

Type A consist of mostly homogenous copact bone, Type B thick layer of compact bone surrounding a core of dense trabecular bone, Type C is a thin layer of cortical bone surrounding a core of dense trabecular bone, and Type D thin layer of cortical bone with a core of low density of trabecular bone (Figs 3.2A to D).

General Health

A review of literature indicates that patients having a variety of systemic conditions may be successfully treated with dental implants, with certain precaution.

Age

Minimum age should be preferred for implants in patients after completion of there growth. Completion of growth is usually earlier in females than males. There is no upper age limit to implant placement, as long as the patient is fit and able to undergo the necessary surgery.

Radiotherapy

Success rates of dental implants are lower in patients with history of radiotherapy compared to non-irradiated patients.

Surgical Techniques

Operative Conditions

Implant surgery should be performed under highly controlled conditions. Contamination of the implant surface during surgical placement should be avoided. Possible sources of contamination from nontitanium surgical instruments and the patient's saliva will have a negative effect on osseointegration.

Incision Technique

A number of different incision types have been advocated, these will be considered for successful implants.

Drilling Technique

Frictional heat during any phase of the drilling procedure will cause a rise in temperature. The critical time/temperature parameter for bone tissue necrosis is around 47°C for one minute. Generation of heat can be kept to a minimum by the use of sharp drills, slow drill speeds, graduated drill sizes and copious water-cooling.

Healing and Loading Time

Delayed Loading

This tried and tested approach involves the implant not being loaded following placement until approximately six months in the maxilla and four months in the mandible. The difference in timing is primarily related to the difference in bone quality between maxilla and mandible.

Early Loading

A number of implant systems with roughened thread designs are considered to be appropriate for early loading within six weeks of implant placement. Such implants should be placed in good quality bone and under favorable circumstances.

Immediate Loading

In certain cases it has been suggested that it may be possible to consider the immediate loading of implants. Factors such as initial implant fit, quality and quantity of available bone, length and diameter of implant, occlusal factors and experience of the operator should be taken into consideration.

CHAPTER
4

Implant Biomaterials

INTRODUCTION

The predicable long-term success of implant-supported prosthesis and other advantages made dental implants the best treatment alternative; several biomaterials are in the scenario today for the fabrication of dental implants such as metals and alloys, ceramics and other synthetic polymers. A number of properties including-ultimate tensile strength, elastic modulus, microstructural phases, grain size, corrosion performance, and biocompatibility are relevant to the proper selection of an alloy for a given clinical problem. Titanium and its alloy, Ti-6Al-4V are the most commonly used biomaterials of the present day due to their unique characteristics. Present chapter briefs, classification of implants and metallurgical aspects as well as the biomechanical properties of titanium and its alloy Ti-6Al-4V, which are needful for the dental implant application.

IMPLANT PROPERTIES

For used in clinical situation some properties of implant biomaterials such as elastic modulus, tensile strength and ductility are used to aid in the design and fabrication of the prosthesis. For example, the elastic modulus of the implant is inversely related to the transmitted force across the implant-tissue interface. An implant with a comparable elastic modulus to bone should be selected to produce a more uniform stress distribution across the interface. Metals possess high strength and ductility, whereas the ceramics and carbons are brittle materials. Ductility is also important because it relates to the potential for permanent deformation of abutments or fixtures in areas of high tensile stress.

CLASSIFICATION OF IMPLANTS MATERIALS

Metals:
- Stainless steel
- Cobalt-chromium-molybdenum based
- Titanium and its alloys
- Surface-coated titanium.

Ceramics:
- Hydroxy apatite
- Bioglass
- Aluminum oxide
- Polymers and composites
- Others gold, carbon, etc.

The major groups of implantable materials in dentistry are metals and alloys, ceramics and polymeric materials.

Most of the dental implantation systems available to date are fabricated from metal or alloys. Metals tested for implants include gold, platinum, palladium, iridium, silver, lead, zinc, aluminum, copper and magnesium. However, they were progressively discontinued from use.

The need for strong corrosion resistant, biocompatible metals brought stainless steel into picture in 1926 and cobalt-chromium-molybdenum-carbon alloys in 1930s.

Stainless steel used in form of surgical austenitic steel, these metals have 18 percent chromium for corrosion resistance and 8 percent nickel to stabilize the austenitic structure. The stainless steel is not used in implant dentistry despite its low cost and ease of fabrication, it was discontinued because of their galvanic potentials and corrosion characteristics (crevice and pitting corrosion).

The cobalt-chromium alloys generally consist of 63 percent cobalt, 30 percent chromium and 5 percent molybdenum with small amount of carbon, manganese, and nickel are discontinued as these alloys exhibit the least ductility of all the alloys systems used for surgical implants.

Some studies raised concerns about galvanic corrosion, studied the local tissue response to stainless steel and cobalt-chromium molybdenum alloys and showed the release of metal ions in the tissues.

Polymeric implants in the form of polymethylmethacrylate and polytetrafluoroethylene were first used in 1930s. The low mechanical strength of the polymers has precluded their use as implants materials because of their susceptibility for mechanical fracture during function.

Titanium, as implant material was investigated extensively in 1960s by Branemark and his associates who established beyond doubt its biocompatibility, besides discovering the process of "osseointegration", which results in direct implant to bone interface. Titanium and its alloys were researched extensively in 1960s but came into increased use from 1970s. After the study the reaction of rabbit to 54 different implanted metals alloys which showed that titanium allowed bone growth directly adjacent to oxide surfaces. Maximum passivity for titanium is reported. Titanium oxidizes (passivates) upon contact with room temperature air and normal tissue fluids. This reactivity is favorable for dental implant devices. This characteristic is one important property for consideration related to the use of titanium for dental implants (Figs 4.1A to C).

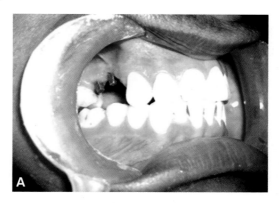

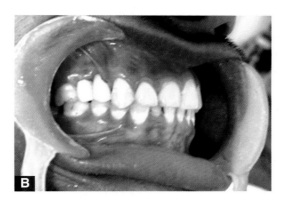

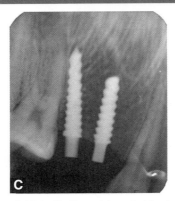

Figs 4.1A to C: Osseointegrated implants

Composition of CP Titanium and Alloys (Weight Percent):

Titanium	N	C	H	Fe	O	Al	V	Ti
CP Grade I	0.03	0.08	0.013	0.20	0.18	—	—	Balance
CP Grade II	0.03	0.08	0.015	0.30	0.25	—	—	Balance
CP Grade III	0.05	0.08	0.015	0.30	0.35	—	—	Balance
CP Grade IV	0.05	0.08	0.015	0.50	0.40	—	—	Balance
Ti-6Al-4V Alloy	0.05	0.08	0.015	0.30	0.20	5.50-6.75	3.50-4.50	Balance
Ti-6Al-4V (ELI alloy)	0.05	0.08	0.012	0.25	0.13	5.50-6.50	3.50-4.50	Balance

Titanium has many favorable properties:
- Low specific gravity
- High heat resistance
- High strength comparable to stainless steel
- Resistant to corrosion
- Modulus of elasticity is closure to the bone.

Most commonly used titanium products are pure titanium and titanium alloys Ti-6Al-4V (names are given according to percentage of approximately 6 percent of Aluminum and 4 percent of Vanadium). Aluminum used for increasing strength and decreasing mass. Vanadium, copper and palladium are used to decrease its susceptibility to corrosion. Titanium alloys are able to maintain that fine balance between sufficient strength to resist fracture under occlusal forces and lower modulus of elasticity for more uniform stress distribution across the bone-implant interface (Fig. 4.2).

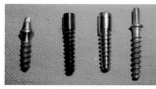

Single piece transgingival
implants

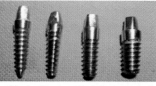

Single piece root form transgingival
implants for immediate placement

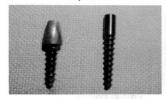

Single piece mini-implant for
overdenture

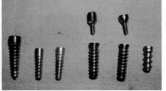

Two piece transgingival and
submerged type implants

Fig. 4.2: Dental implants of different types fabricated from CP titanium

The date multinational survey by ISO (International Organization for Standardization) has indicated that titanium and its alloys are mainly used for dental implants. The metal titanium acquired the name "Wonder Metal" due to a unique combination of several useful properties like its exceptional corrosion/erosion resistance, good fatigue and fatigue toughness, biocompatibility. Selecting an alloy with the best physical, chemical and biological properties should be the main criteria for a specific clinical situation.

Biocompatibility

It is ability of material to perform with an appropriate response in a specific application. Biocompatibility is affected by the intrinsic nature of the material, as well as its design and construction. Therefore the state of biocompatibility may be confined to a particular situation or function in the human body. Some acceptance provision of implant material as follows:

• Evaluation of physical properties
• Ease of fabrication and sterilization potential without material degradation
• Metal toxicity and biological acceptability
• Freedom from defects
• A few clinical trials.

Metal toxicity and biological acceptability can be studies *in vitro* and *in vivo* environments, using the following tests:

1. Hemolysis test
2. Mast cell degranulation

3. Cell death in tissue culture
4. Skin and mucous membrane sensitization
5. Osseous tissue response in animals, e.g. canines
6. Human clinical trials.

The property of biocompatibility of metals is by their passivating oxide film of semi or non-conductive nature, which prevents the exchange of electrons and the resultant flow of ions within the adjacent tissues, which is injurious to cellular activity. It is not only demands a passive film, but also a resistant film. The film should have low solubility in the body fluid. Titanium outscores other metals in the formation of a resistant and passive oxide film.

Response of the bone to different implant materials is the principal factor on which an implant biomaterial is selected as suitable or unsuitable for osseointegration. Reports have concluded that the percentage of bone volume in cortical bone around CPTi and HA implants were the same. However when it is placed in bone marrow, a marked difference was reported. This clearly emphasizes the need for more studies highlighting the effects of biomaterials to surrounding tissues as well their effect on clinical effectiveness.

Biofunctionality (Elastic Modulus)

It has been desired that the inserted biomaterial have isoelasticity (similar to modulus of elasticity) to that of its host system (bone). Some scientist discussed the engineering aspects of isoelasticity. They state that, if a close bone contact has to be achieved and maintained, the bond at the bone-implant must be strong to withstand all shear forces. Isoelasticity results in similar deformation patterns on loading in implant and bone, preventing shear forces at implant host tissue "osseointegration" interface.

Modulus of elasticity of pure titanium and Ti-6Al-4V is closure to that of bone than any other widely used implant material. This ensures a more uniform distribution of stress, particularly along the bone-implant interface, as the bone and the implant flex similarly.

Bio-adhesion

Bony apposition plays a vital role for rigid fixation of metallic implants. However, since the dental implants traverse three different types of tissues, creating three interfaces, these being epithelial attachment, connective tissue interface and bone tissue interface, thus requiring different surface characterization of the implant. With the use of newer implantation techniques, implant site can be prepared such that the interviewing soft fibrous tissue may be avoided, to further improve and to achieve perfect integration. The implant is left unloaded during an initial critical period of 3-4 weeks. Surface characterization, to improve bony in growth into the rougher surface and to have a better bone volume ratio (BVR) can be achieved by porous coating, electro discharge compaction, plasma spraying, chemical etching, sand blasting and other similar methods.

THE IMPLANT SURFACE AND COATING (SURFACE MODIFICATION)

The titanium implant surface is processed to make the surface bioactive and to increase the surface area for stable bone-implant interface.

Brief Overview Over Surface Modification

Surface modification consists of various techniques where we alter the surface properties of the metal. Surface modification can be mechanical, e.g. (grit blasting), chemical (alkali or acid) treatment, electroplating (with gold, etc.), coupling agents (silane reagents), plasma spraying, anodization (to form porous barriers), newer techniques like the use of lasers.

Why Do We Need Surface Modification?

We need surface treatment either to:
- Remove surface contaminants that may have been incorporated during manufacturing
- After the surface chemistry of the metal so as to bring better bonding between the metal and adherent
- Increase surface roughness of the metal which increases the surface area which is used for bonding
- To increase the corrosion resistance of the parent metal
- To make the metal passive.

Techniques of Surface Modification of Titanium

1. *Anodization:* Pure titanium has ability to form several oxides, including TiO, Ti_2O_3, TiO_2. Of

these, TiO_2 is considered the most stable and is used more often under physiological conditions. It acts as a potential barrier for foreign bodies to directly attack the surface of titanium. Thus titanium does not corrode easily.

2. *Hydroxyapatite coating:* Major portion of our bone consists of hydroxyapatite. When we put titanium implants into the bone, the time take for osseointegration is more. So, in order to make a better bonding between the implant surface and bone, we apply hydroxyapatite coating on the surface of titanium so that body accept it in a more natural way and the healing period is less. With the help of this technique we can load the implant at a shorter time, thus saving the time for edentulous patient together with better results.

3. *Surface modification of titanium by plasma nitriding:* The use of commercially pure titanium as implant material poses a threat to long time survival due to its low wear resistance. In dentistry when an implant is placed it has to be kept clean, some people try using Gracy scalers, which may damage the implant surface. A suitable alternative to overcome this problem is plasma nitriding where we treat sample with 80 percent N_2 and 20 percent H_2 at temperature of 600°C to 800°C. The results seem to increase the tribiological properties of commercially pure titanium.

4. *Polyethylene grafted polycationic polymers* can be added to the surface of titanium. PEG polymers gets bonded to negatively changed TiO_2 which later helps surface proteins to bond with the surface modified titanium implants. Better

natural healing environment can be created with the help of this method.

5. *Alkali treatment of titanium surface:* Commercially pure titanium samples are taken and are treated with alkali. The alkali treatment created a porous, hydrated and reactive titanium oxide surface. The contact angle of the alkali treated sample was seen to be decreased than non treated samples. With the help of this treatment we can do early bonding of the implant. The healing period of alkali treated implants was seen to be 50 percent less than the conventional implants.

6. *Lasers:* An advantage of lasers in surface modification is that laser has the property of melting surface layer locally, as in practice wear is often restricted to specific area. In addition laser processing is contact less and the thermal mechanical deformation of the substrate is generally low. Following types of lasers are used.

- CO_2 lasers
- Nd-YAG laser

To embed a new phase in a substrate by means of laser processing the new material can be pre-positioned on the substrate. However, to melt the substrate the heat has to be transported through the pre-positioned powder slurry. If the melting point of both the materials does not differ to a large extent, a reasonable degree of mixture may occur. If this is undesirable, the possibility of powder injection should be considered.

SELECTION OF AN IMPLANT MATERIAL

Since abundance of different implant materials and implant systems, it is important to know the indications for use of these different materials. Strength, types of bone, implant design, abutment choices and availability, surface finish, and biomechanical considerations are important factors for selection of implant materials:

- Strength of an implant is often a consideration, depending on the area of placement of the implant. If the implants are located in a high load zone (e.g. in the posterior areas of the arch) the clinician might consider using higher strength material such as CP grade IV titanium or one of titanium alloys. Some controversy exists as to which titanium metal to use, because some researchers believe that aluminum and vanadium can be toxic if released in sufficient quantities

- Other considerations for selection include a history of implant fracture in the placement area of interest, the use of narrower implants, and history of occlusal or parafunctional habits. Anterior implants designated for use in narrow spaces have smaller diameter in the range of 3.25 mm. Conversely, single implants placed in posterior areas have larger diameters up to 5 mm

- Type of bone in which the implant will be placed is of critical importance

- There is much debate about when to use metal implants or ceramic coated implants. Current review suggests that the survival rates are similar for both coated and uncoated implants and that the HA-coating did not compromise the long-term survival of these implants. Indications to support the selection of hydroxyapatite coated implants

over titanium or metallic surfaced implants include:
- The need for greater bone-implant interface contact area
- The ability to place the implants in type IV bone,
- Fresh extraction sites, and
- Newly grafted sites.

It has also been shown that the advantage of HA-coated implants are mainly short-term in nature and are related to the initial stability of the implant, which most often determines its prerestorative success or failure.

BIOMECHANICS

The attachment of bone to implants serves as the basis for the biomechanics analyses performed for dental implants. Close approximation of osseo-integrated bone with surface of an implant fixture permits the transfer of stresses with little relative displacement of the bone and implant. The stresses that are generated are highly affected by three main variables:
- Masticatory forces-frequency, bite force, and mandibular movements
- Support for prosthesis-implant supported, implant-tissue supported, implant-tooth supported
- The mechanical properties of materials involved in the implant prosthesis or restoration.

One of the most important variables affecting the close apposition of bone to the implant surface is the relative movement or "micromotion". It has long been documented that movement shortly after implantation prevents the formation of the bone and encourages the formation of fibrous connective tissue around implant surface. This collagen rich connective tissue is considered to be nonretentive and provides no support for the implant fixture. This is the reason that a delay of 4-6 months is recommended before loading after surgery. There has been some success reported with immediate loading of implants depending on bone quality and patient selection.

The type of restoration based on the initial Branemark hybrid prosthesis for the atrophic mandible (Figs 4.3A to C) usually involves 4-6 implant fixture confined to the area between the mental foramina of the mandible with cantilevers extending from the most distal implant. These were restored with acrylic resin and denture teeth, which were attached to the implant metal superstructure through the use of chemical and mechanical bonding.

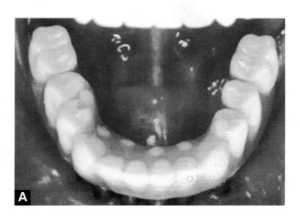

A

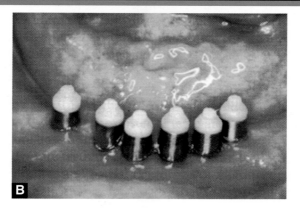

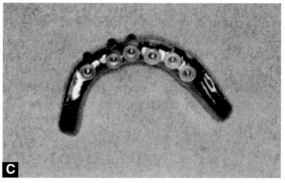

Figs 4.3A to C: (A) The original Branemark hybrid prosthesis designed to accommodate severely atrophic mandibles (B) The hybrid prosthesis usually requires 4 to 6 implants (C) Corresponding superstructure that is screwed onto the implants

When two or more implants are placed in straight line, the bending moment will be distributed proportionately to all fixtures, provided the prosthesis is sufficiently rigid.

- Placement of implants in an offset manner has been suggested as a more favorable orientation because it is believed to increase the resistance to loading
- Wider diameter implants placed in a straight line minimize more stresses as compare to tripodization of implants
- Load is greatest at the most distal fixture when an anteriorly positioned cantilever prosthesis is exists. Thus the distance between the most terminal abutment and one directly adjacent to it should be increased to reduce the stress and strain induced within the most distal abutment
- An inaccurate fit will lead to a nonuniform distribution of load with the unit closest to the load bearing most of the forces
- The Branemark hybrid implants have been designed with variable cantilever distances based on number of implants available in the prosthesis. Branemark recommended a maximum length of three premolars. Others recommended a 15-20 mm separation in the mandible and 10 mm in the maxilla because of poor bone quality. Any cantilever length over 7 mm causes the largest increases in microstrain within both framework and bone
- As far as possible the attachment of implants to natural teeth should be avoided and that having, lone standing implants is a better restorative option unless it is absolutely necessary to include a natural tooth in the restoration. Although some of previous studies suggest that the attachment

of natural teeth to implants does not compromise the prognosis of the prosthesis

- Several devices such as the IMZ intramobile element have been developed to allow the implant to accommodate the movement of the periodontal ligament (Fig. 4.4).

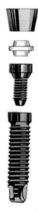

Fig. 4.4: Intramobile element that is believed to act as an internal shock absorber

CONCLUSION

The implant systems currently available are diverse. Titanium and its alloys do wonders in the hands of the dentist. Discovery of its properties for the usage as dental implant materials has revolutionized the implantology in world. Commercially pure titanium (Cp Titanium) and Ti-6Al-4V are commonly used and latest titanium niobium alloy is under study. Apart from titanium, extensive research is going on towards the development of bioceramics and synthetic polymers and other biomaterials. When the mechanisms that ensure implant bioacceptance and structural stabilization are fully understood, implant failure will become a rare occurrence, provided that they are used properly and placed in sites for which they are indicated.

CHAPTER
5

Case Selection

The Goal of modern dentistry is to return patients to oral health in a predictable fashion. The partial and complete edentulous patient may be unable to recover normal function, esthetics, comfort, or speech with a traditional removable prosthesis. Implant prosthesis often offer a more predictable treatment option than traditional restorations.

REASONS FOR TOOTH LOSS

The reason for the loss of the tooth must be ascertained, as this can be influence treatment planning. The prognosis of dentition as a whole and prognosis of the teeth adjacent to the space must be determined. Depending on the nature of the dental disease and ease of tooth extraction there will be a variable degree of soft and hard tissue loss once the teeth have been removed. With implants tissue loss should be minimal, but in severe cases of tissue loss a compromised result may occur unless some form of augmentation is considered.

Main reasons for tooth loss or missing teeth are as follows:

Periodontal Diseases

Patient having advanced type of periodontal diseases, conventional tooth and implant abutments may be equally at risk from future bone loss. With dental implants some form of soft tissue or bone augmentation is typically required (Fig. 5.1).

Dental Caries

Dental caries weakens tooth structure. Treatment of dental caries with plastic or cast restorations

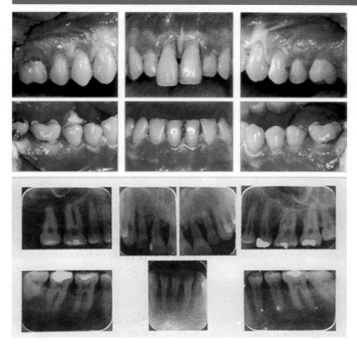

Fig. 5.1: Localized, aggressive periodontitis (molars and incisiors)

results in further loss of tooth structure, and progression of caries with further destruction may be required endodontic treatment followed by the need for auxiliary retention by means of pins or posts. The potential for early failure of heavily restored teeth makes treatment-planning uncertain.

Endodontic Failure

Endodontic treatment is generally successful. When endodontic failure occurs repeat treatments may suffer limitations. It is useful to fully asses the expected prognosis of such teeth and carry out a cost/benefit analysis of retreating them. Often it may be more appropriate to consider removal and replacement of the tooth rather than attempting a repair or replacement restoration.

Trauma

Severe trauma may lead to hard and soft tissue loss. Teeth may be avulsed or fractured. It is often difficult to predict the prognosis of traumatized teeth. A significant proportion of such teeth lose their vitality perhaps 5-10 years after the initial trauma. This reduces their ability to perform as potential abutments for bridges or dentures. Traumatized teeth can be affected by internal and external resorption.

Hypodontia

Approximately 6 percent of population is affected by hypodontia or congenital absence of teeth, which also includes patient with cleft lip and palate or other craniofacial anomalies. Where teeth are missing, the alveolar ridge is often narrow and wasted. This complicates orthodontic treatment and subsequent tooth replacement.

REPLACEMENT OF MISSING TEETH

The reasons for replacing teeth include:
* To improve appearance
* To improve function
* Maintenance of oral health.

Following an extraction, there is always the possibility of teeth tilting or drifting into edentulous space within the same dental arch. Similarly, if occlusion is unstable the opposing teeth may erupt into the edentulous space. It has been observed that food packing, dental caries, occlusal abnormalities and temporomandibular joint (TMJ) dysfunction and other dental conditions have ensued following adverse tooth movements. Conversely, it has been shown that, if such movements have not occurred within 5 years of a tooth extraction, it is unlikely they will occur in the future. Therefore, if it is decided not to replace lost tooth immediately the situation should be reviewed for periods of up to 5 years before the edentulous space can be considered stable.

Patients have their own individual smile. This generally includes all anterior teeth and in some extreme cases the molar teeth. If smile-line is generous and there is an excessive show of gingiva, dentist understandably becomes more concern about providing a solution to missing teeth.

The enjoyment and efficiency of mastication is severely reduced when multiple teeth are missing. It is subjective decision by the patient as to whether he or she has sufficient teeth to enjoy food. Both the dentist and the patient must be convinced of the need for tooth replacement before treatment options are considered.

Options for Replacement of Teeth for the Partially Dentate Case

It is important, that treatment with dental implants viewed in the context of overall patient care, and as one of a range of procedures that may be used to help the patient. Complex therapy is not inherently superior and simpler procedures may, in many situations be more appropriate. Various options regarding various restorative procedures and wide range of alternative approaches to the management of tooth loss must be considered in the best interest of the patient.

No Replacement

It should not be assumed that the absence of teeth is an absolute indication for their replacement, which should confer clear benefits.

Systemic Factors

A patient who has a very poor residual life expectancy may have little wish to receive extensive dental treatment, and prefer to have problems managed as they arise. In these situations implant procedures would be inappropriate—

- There is some patient for whom restoration of missing teeth is a low priority
- When patient is unable to attend for a care for reasons of ill health or family or work or commitments then little treatment may be feasible
- Some patients suffer from systemic problems that severely limit their ability to co-operate with treatment.

Local Factors

These relate to oral status and the requirement to prepare a long-term plan for oral health commensurate with patient's needs and wishes. This will involve an assessment of their oral status, the function of the dentition and expected benefits of any possible treatment.

Orthodontic Management

This is not available as an option owing to technical problems or lack of suitable teeth to move into defect. However, in appropriate cases it can be a valuable method of eliminating a space in the arch. It has also a role in facilitating implant treatment by realigning teeth adjacent to potential implant sites, so, as to make the space a more suitable size for placing the implants supporting a suitable crown. This is relevant not only for the edentulous span but also for the alignment of the roots of adjacent teeth.

Removable Partial Dentures

Treatment with removable partial dentures is an extremely versatile procedure, which is widely used in the management of partial tooth loss, both as an interim measure and as the definitive treatment. Correctly utilized and supported by thorough oral hygiene and maintenance, it has minimal harmful effects on the oral cavity.

Adhesive Bridges

The development of adhesive technique has made it possible to restore many edentulous spaces with resin bonded bridges, which can provide a very satisfactory replacement with minimal tooth preparation.

Conventional Bridges

Prior to development of reliable adhesive techniques in dentistry, conventional bridges were often considered the ideal treatment for restoration of partially dentate arch. Extensive tooth preparation is one of the disadvantages.

Implant Stabilized Prosthesis

This is a complex technique, which can be used to stabilize both fixed and removable prosthesis and one which reduces the rate of resorption of alveolar bone. One of the main advantages of using dental implants is that they can replace teeth without involving natural tooth abutments (Fig. 5.2). It is technically demanding and unsuited to many clinical situations.

General Considerations

1. Patient must be medically fit to undergo surgery and complex prosthodontic treatment over multiple visits (caution with uncontrolled diabetics, irradiated bone, coagulation problems, smokers have much higher failure rate, high dose steroids).
2. The bony implant site should be of sufficient height, width and quality for implant placement.
3. The implant site must not impinge on key anatomical features such as maxillary sinus, mental foramen, etc.
4. Implant must be placed in such a manner so that they can be restored esthetically and functionally.

Dental Considerations

1. Patient should be able to maintain good oral hygiene.

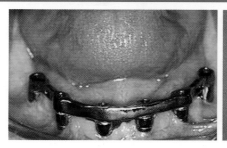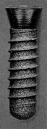

Fig. 5.2: Implants placement for fixed prosthesis

2. Pre-existing periodontal disease and caries should be controlled.
3. There should be enough inter ridge space for implant superstructures and prosthesis (minimum 7 mm).
4. There should be enough space between existing teeth for implant placement without tooth damage (7 mm).

Clinical examination of future implant site helps to evaluate:

- Amount of attached mucosa
- Amount of bone
- Unfavorable frenum or high muscle attachment.

Dental implants may be treatment of choice in the following situations:

- Unrestored dentition
- Heavily restored dentition (failed bridgework)
- Spaced dentition
- Lack of suitable abutments (microdont teeth and lack of tooth structure)
- Problematic denture wearer (poor anatomy and gag reflex).

Similarly there are circumstances where, it is difficult or inappropriate to consider dental implants.
- Poor prognosis dentition
- Lack of interdental space (lower anterior teeth)
- Lack of interocclusal space
- Young patient who have not completed growth.

SUMMARY

Dentures and bridges should always be considered as alternative approach for tooth replacement. Orthodontist can close some spaces. Implants are the treatment of choice for most edentulous spaces. Soft and hard tissue loss will compromise the appearances unless augmentation is considered. Prognosis of individual teeth and the whole dentition needs to be estimated.

CHAPTER
6

Implant Placement in Patients having Systemic Disorders

Implant therapy can greatly improve the function and esthetics of carefully selected partially or completely edentulous patients. Before any form of implant therapy is considered in any patient, the medical history must be thoroughly reviewed and if appropriate, a physical examination performed. An existing systemic disease or ongoing systemic therapy may complicate or contraindicate implant dentistry. An increased knowledge of the underlying disease process has improved the management of the patients suffering from bone metabolism abnormalities, diabetes mellitus, xerostomia and ectodermal dysplasias.

METABOLIC BONE DISEASE

Bone mass depends on the equilibrium between bone formation and resorption within a remodeling unit, as well as on the number of remodeling units activated within a given period of time in a defined area of bone.

When bone resorption exceeds bone formation, that will results in decrease in bone mass or osteoporosis (metabolic disease). Various case reports given by various implantologists have indicated that implants can be successfully placed in osteoporotic patients.

- Prior to implant surgery, a careful assessment of nutrition and systemic health in patients at risk for metabolic bone disease is recommended
- Patients should undergo an endocrinologic, orthopedic, or obstetric examination and be treated, if necessary. Physiologic doses of vitamin D (from 400 to 800 IU/day) and calcium

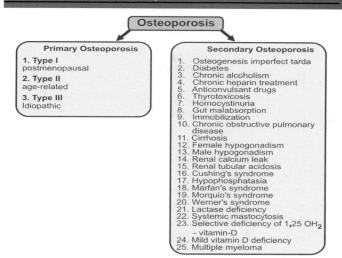

are recommended during the postoperative period. In all cases a balanced preoperative and post-operative diet should be recommended

- Patient should attempt to give up smoking, since smoking is an important risk factor for osteoporosis and implant failure
- In cases of insufficient bone volume, the implant sites should be augmented before or during implant surgery
- The occlusal load should be properly distributed throughout the dentition to avoid overloading the implant which may contribute to implant loss.
- The healing period should be extended, before construction of prosthodontic appliance
- Preference should be given to implant designs that will have close bone-implant contact on insertion to ensure primary stabilization in less dense osteoporotic bone.

Pre and Intraoperative Considerations
- Examination of causative factors for bone disease and treatment
- Bone augmentation if necessary

Postoperative Considerations and Maintenance
- Physiological doses of vitamin D (400-800 IU/day) and calcium (1500 mg/day) during the postoperative period
- The healing period should be increased by 2 months to 8 months in the maxilla and 6 months in the mandible
- Careful occlusal adjustment and careful examination for signs of occlusal overload, e.g. bruxism

DIABETES MELLITUS

Analysis of the epidemiological data regarding diabetes mellitus indicates that all dentists will encounter patients with diabetes mellitus and that clinicians who perform intraoral surgery such as implant placement should have a thorough knowledge of this disease. In the oral cavity, diabetes mellitus is associated with xerostomia, increased levels of salivary glucose, swelling of parotid gland, and an increased incidence of caries and periodontitis as well as other infection of the oral cavity. Although dental implant therapy seems to be a helpful tool in restoring the dental status of diabetic patients, it appears prudent for clinicians to adhere to the following guidelines (Fig. 6.1).

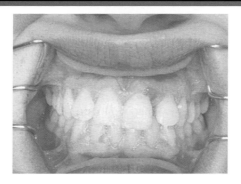

Fig. 6.1: Gingivitis in diabetic patients

- Proper antibiotic prophylaxis is recommended
- To use chlorhexidine rinses peri and post-operatively at the time of implant placement

---

Pre and Intraoperative Considerations
- Metabolic control should be analyzed and optimized prior to implant surgery if not sufficient. A glycosylated hemoglobin level near 7 mg/percent is advisable
- Antibiotic prophylaxis is recommended
- Peri and postoperative rinse with 0.12 percent chlorhexidine digluconate

Postoperative Considerations and Maintenance
- Shorten recall intervals to detect intraoral infectious disease

Hydroxyapatite plasma-spray-coated implants have been found to have a higher survival rate than titanium implants in diabetic patients. Poorly controlled diabetic patients are more difficult to manage, and delay in surgery is recommended until better control is achieved. The placement of dental implants in patient with metabolically controlled diabetes appears to be successful as in the general population.

XEROSTOMIA

There are numerous pathologic conditions, that are accompanied by reduced salivary flow
- Therapeutic head and neck irradiation
- Autoimmune diseases (Sjögren's syndrome, systemic lupus erythematosus, etc.)
- Infectious disease such as HIV and hepatitis C
- Diabetes mellitus
- Drugs-antihistamines diuretics, tricyclic anti-depressants, etc.

Xerostomia or reduced salivary flow causes bacterial infection, fungal infection and adverse effect on successful prosthetic reconstruction especially removable dentures.

Prior to implant placement, the underlying cause of the xerostomia needs to be properly diagnosed and treated. Any oral bacterial infections such as periodontitis, caries, or fungal infections such as candidiasis should be thoroughly treated prior to implant placement. After implant placement, maintenance interval should be shortened to prevent the development of peri-implantitis due to

Water/metabolite loss	**Interference with neural transmission**
• Impaired water intake	• Medications/drugs
• Blood loss	• Autonomic dysfunction (e.g. ganglionic
• Loss of water to skin (fever, burns,   neuropathia)
excessive sweating)	• Conditions affecting the CNS (e.g.
• Emesis	Alzheimer´s disease)
• Diarrhea	• Psychogenic disorders (depression,
• Renal water loss	anxiety)
• Polyuria (diabetes insipidus)	• Trauma
• Osmotic diuresis (diabetes mellitus)	• Decrease in mastication

Xerostomia

Damage to the salivary glands	Protein caloric malnutrition
• Therapeutic irradiation to the head and neck region	
• Autoimmune diseases (primary or secondary Sjögren's syndrome, graft-versus-host disease, systemic lupus erythematosus, rheumatoid arthritis, etc.)	
• Infectious diseases (HIV, hepatitis, etc.)	
• Ageing (?)	

the increased plaque formation in these patients. Stimulation of salivary flow can be achieved by either physiological (sugar free chewing gum) or pharmacological (cholinergic agonist, e.g. pilocarpin and cevimeline).

Pre and Intraoperative Considerations
- Treatment of bacterial or fungal intraoral infections
- Increase salivary flow

Postoperative Considerations and Maintenance
- Shorten recall intervals to detect infection

ECTODERMAL DYSPLASIA

Ectodermal dysplasia (ED) represent a rare group of inherited disorders that occur in approximately 1 per

100,000 live births. Ectodermal dysplasia is characterized by the classical tried of hypodontia, hypohydrosis and hypotrichosis and characteristic features such as prominent supraorbital ridges, frontal bossing, and a depressed nasal bridge (Fig. 6.2).

Principal aims of dental treatment are to restore missing teeth and bone, establish a normal vertical dimension and provide support for the facial soft tissues. Conventional prosthodontic treatment (complete dentures, overdentures, or a combination of bridge work and removable partial dentures) often faces severe problems due to anatomical abnormalities of existing teeth and alveolar ridges resulting in poor retention and instability of prosthesis. The short coming of removable prosthesis furthermore includes dental hygiene problems, speech difficulties, and dietary limitations. Moreover, progressive resorption of basal bone when the edentulous ridge is loaded at an early age may even aggravate the problem.

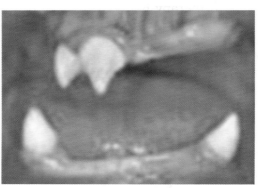

Fig. 6.2: Hypodontia and cone shaped teeth in ectodermal dysplasia

Pre and Intraoperative Considerations

- Whenever possible postpone implantation until skeletal and dental growth has been completed
- If implant therapy is necessary in the maxilla: divide prosthetic bar attachments that cross the maxillary midline

Postoperative Considerations and Maintenance

- Shorten recall intervals to detect infectious disease
- Careful examination for possible movements of the implant due to growth of the jaws
- Adapt prosthetics to growth-induced changes

- Whenever possible postpone implantation until skeletal and dental growth has been completed
- If implant therapy is necessary in the maxilla: divide prosthetic bar attachments that cross the maxillary midline
- If implant therapy is necessary in the mandible: implant placement should be done in the anterior mandible
- Shorten recall intervals to detect infectious disease
- Careful examination for possible movements of the implant placement due to growth of the jaws
- Adapt prosthesis to growth induced changes.

CARDIOVASCULAR DISORDERS

Hypertension

- Essential hypertension is treated with medications, many of which have impact on

implant therapy because of their numerous side effects
- A medication such as flurazepam 30 mg or diazepam 5 to 10 mg may be prescribed in the evening to help the patient sleep quietly in the night before the procedure
- Blood pressure above 160/100 should be referred to a physician for medical management.

Angina Pectoris

Angina pectoris or chest pain in the cardiac muscle is a form of coronary heart disease. Etiology is transient myocardial oxygen demand in excess of supply. Classical retrosternal pain develops due to stress and physical exertion, radiates to shoulder, left arm, mandible, neck, palate and tongue. These symptoms are relieved by rest and duration of episode is about 3 to 5 minutes.

Dental emergency kit should include nitroglycerine tablets (0.3 to 0.4 mg) or a translingual spray, which is to be replaced every 6 months. During an attack all dental treatment is stopped immediately, nitroglycerine is administered sublingually with 100 percent oxygen at 6 lt/min. If patient is not relieved within 8 to 10 minutes, patient is transported to a hospital.

Patients with mild angina attack (One attack/month) can undergo most nonsurgical dental procedure with normal protocol. Advanced restorative procedures and minor implant surgery is done with nitrous oxide sedation. Appointment should be as short as possible; this may require more than one surgical or restorative appointment. Use of vasoconstrictors should be limited.

Myocardial Infarction

Myocardial infarction is prolonged ischemia or lack of oxygen that causes injury to the heart. The patient usually complains of severe chest pain in pericardial or substernal region. Dental evaluation should include the dates of all episodes of MI, especially the latest and any complications. Medical consultation should preclude any extensive restorative and surgical procedure. Longer procedures should be segmented into several shorter appointments. Elective implant should be at least postponed for 12 months following MI.

Congestive Heart Failure (CHF)

Congestive heart failure is a chronic heart condition in which heart is failing as a pump. Symptoms of CHF include abnormal tiredness or shortness of breadth (DYSPNEA) brought on by slight activity or even occurring at rest(these symptoms are due to excess fluid in lungs and partly due to excess work required of the heart), wheezing caused by fluids in lungs (pulmonary edema), peripheral edema or swelling of the ankles (pedal edema) and lower legs, frequent urination at night, jugular venous distention sounds at auscultation, and paroxysmal nocturnal dyspnea, sensation of unable to breathe, which may interrupt sleep.

A lethal dose of digitalis is only twice the treatment dose. The dentist who recognizes the more common side effects should report them to treating physician. Patients on digoxican and diuretics should have serum electrolytes evaluated before surgery to check imbalances.

Subacute Bacterial Endocarditis (SABE)/ Valvular Heart Disease

Bacterial endocarditis is an infection of the heart valves or endothelial surfaces of the heart. Dental procedures causing transient bacterimia are a major cause of bacterial endocarditis. Implant dentist should be familiar with antibiotic regimens for heart conditions requiring prophylaxis. In some patient with a limited oral hygiene potential implant therapy may be contraindicated because of high risk of endocarditis.

THYROID DISORDERS

The major function of thyroid is production of hormone thyroxin (T_4). Thyroxin is responsible for the regulation of carbohydrate, protein and lipid metabolism. In addition hormone potentiates the action of other hormone such as catecholamines and growth hormones. Patients with hyperthyroidism are extremely sensitive to catecholamines such as epinephrine in local anesthetics and gingival retraction cords. When exposure to catecholamines is coupled with stress (often related with dental procedure) and tissue damage (Implant surgery) an exacerbation of the symptoms of hyperthyroidism can occur. Hypothyroid patient is sensitive to CNS depressant drugs; such as diazepam and barbiturates. The risk of respiratory depression or cardiovascular depression or collapse, must be considered.

ADRENAL GLAND DISORDERS

The adrenal glands are endocrine organs located just above the kidneys. Epinephrine and norepinephrine are produced by glands, which is responsible for the control of blood pressure, myocardial contractility and excitability, and general metabolism. Glucocorticosteriods secreted by these glands help in decreasing swelling and pain. Addisons disease shows decrease in adrenal function. These patients show weakness, weight loss, orthostatic hypotension, nausea and vomiting. When these signs are noted, implant dentist should require a medical consultation. Cushing's disease describes hyper function in adrenal glands; characteristics changes associated with this disease are moon facies, truncal obesity or buffalo hump, muscle wasting and hirutism. These patients bruise easily, have poor wound healing, experience osteoporosis, and are at increased risk for infection.

Additional steroids are prescribed for the patient just before stressful situation. Patient with known adrenal disorder, physician should be consulted.

PREGNANCY

Implant surgery procedures are contraindicated for the pregnant patient. All elective procedures with the exception of oral prophylaxis should be deferred after childbirth.

HEMATOLOGIC DISEASES

Patient suffering from anemia have bone maturation problem and is impaired in long term anemic patient, basically loss in trabecular pattern of bone which is very important for implant stability. Abnormal bleeding is also common problem of these diseases.

Treatment planning modifications should towards more conservative approach, surgical procedures should be delayed until infection or disease is controlled or returned to a normal condition.

CHRONIC OBSTRUCTIVE PULMONARY DISEASES

Two common forms of obstructive pulmonary diseases are emphysema and chronic bronchitis. The use of epinephrine should be limited. Drugs that depress respiratory function such as sedatives (including nitrous oxide), tranquilizers, and narcotics should be discussed with physician.

LIVER CIRRHOSIS

It occurs as a result of injury to liver cells and progressives scarring. Patient with liver diseases, 50 percent have prolonged PT time and clinical bleeding. The inability to detoxify drugs may result in oversedation or respiratory depression. The laboratory evaluation of implant candidate gives much insight to hepatic function. Elective implant therapy is relative contraindicated in the patient with symptoms of active alcoholism.

VITAMIN D DISORDERS

The deficiency of vitamin D leads to osteomalacia. Implants are not contraindicated, although treatment is same as osteoporotic patient.

HYPERPARATHYROIDISM

Clinical patients develop loose teeth, altered trabecular pattern of bone with ground glass appearance. Implants are not contraindicated if no bony lesions are present in the implant placement region.

FIBROUS DYSPLASIA

Fibrous dysplasia is a disorder in which, fibrous connective tissue replaces areas of normal bone. Implants placement is contraindicated in the regions of this disorder.

TOBACCO

Reports in the literature demonstrate lower success rates for endosteal implants in smokers. Although implants may be placed in patients that smoke, failure rates are quite high in smokers the risk need to be evaluated and carefully explained to the patient. Ideally patient should be discouraged for smoking.

PSYCHOLOGICAL PROBLEMS

The suitability of patients having psychological disorders must be assessed before any implant placement.

SUMMARY

For appraisal of the limits and options of dental implants in the medically compromised patient, additional reliable, clinically relevant, information is needed. Based on sound clinical evidence, more detailed guidelines can be developed that may aid in the improved predictability of dental implants in the special-patient category.

CHAPTER
7

Examination and Treatment Planning

INTRODUCTION

A systemic approach to patient assessment is required. It is carried out in a very similar way to any assessment of a patient needing dental treatment. It is important to obtain a detail medical and clinical assessment before embarking on tooth extraction and starting implant therapy. Suitable patients' education about the benefits of dental implants, motivation and also persuasion to undergo implant therapy is important. The protocol for a successful implant is one that demonstrates osseointegration, as well as optimal position of the implant for the fabrication of an esthetic and functional restoration. Ideal placement facilitates the establishment of favorable forces on the implants and prosthetic components while ensuring an esthetic outcome. To increase the predictability of success, it is essential that the implants are placed in proper patients using proper treatment planning. A well planned treatment planning is critical for implant success. The clinician must determine all the potential risks and the suitability of the patient for an implant supported restoration.

Complete medical examination with detailed history should be carried out to rule out the presence of any systemic disorders. Systemic diseases have a broad effect (details were discussed in previous chapter). They may be categorized as mild, moderate and severe. After patient selection, thorough medical and dental history is taken and examination is carried out.

The medical history includes
• Cardiac disorders
• Endocrine disorders

- Blood disorders
- Bone disorders
- Hepatic disorders
- Allergic reaction to drugs.

It is important to pay particular attention to the following:

- *Smoking:* Although implants may be placed in patients that smoke, although failure rates are quite high in smokers the risk need to be evaluated and carefully explained to the patient. It may disturb osseointegration. Ideally patient should be discouraged for smoking
- *Diabetes:* Uncontrolled diabetes should be stabilized before contemplating implant. Implants can be placed in patients with diabetes if the condition is controlled
- *Facial pain or atypical neuralgia:* The origin of any facial pain needs to be carefully diagnosed. Particular care must be taken with patient suffering from atypical facial pain, as an implant may become a focus for this pain
- *Psychological problems:* The suitability of patients having psychological disorders must be assessed before any implant placement.

Lab investigations to rule out any systemic diseases or bleeding disorders

- Hemoglobin levels, erythrocyte sedimentation rate (ESR)
- Total leukocyte count (TLC), differential leukocyte count (DLC) and platelet count
- Clotting time, and bleeding time
- Bone density (if possible).

Dental history and examination included

- *Extraoral:* It should be carried out, with particular attention being paid to the following:
    i. TMJ and Muscles of mastication are examined for anatomical abnormalities, signs of dysfunction and pathology.
    ii. Facial profile and lip support, with and without any existing denture, needs to be carefully evaluated and atypical features noted.
    iii. *Smile line:* The smile line relates to the level of upper and lower lips in relations to the corresponding gingival margin. It is of particularly importance in cases in which gingival defects and long teeth are included in the smile. A high lip line may be demanding aesthetically.
- *Intraoral:*
    – Recording of the cause and duration of tooth loss
    – Assessment of oral hygiene
    – Oral health
    – Prognosis of remaining teeth
    – Ridge thickness and shape
    – Occlusion
    – Para functional habits
    – Availability of bone
    – Space-interdental and interocclusal.
- *Dental investigations*

ROLE OF STUDY MODELS

After medical and dental check-up, preoperative treatment planning is done. First step is to articulate the study models. This provides informations like

- Occlusal centric relation; any premature occlusal contact
- Edentulous ridge relationship to adjacent teeth and opposing arches
- Interarch space
- Position of adjacent teeth including inclination, rotation, extrusion, spacing, parallelism and esthetic considerations
- Direction of forces in future implant sites
- Diagnostic wax-up is done on study models which is used to fabricate radiographic templates and surgical templates.

It is invariably necessary to obtain articulated study casts to allow a well considered treatment plan to be formulated. Study models should be articulated to assess the occlusal scheme, individual tooth relation, tooth morphology, arch relationship, interarch space and direction of forces on the future implant site. On the articulated study model, diagnostic wax-up will be done.

Diagnostic/Surgical Stent

Diagnostic stent should be fabricated on it with clear acrylic material. The planned implant site will be filled with radiopaque material (for CT scan) and steel sphere placed (for OPG). The diagnostic stents must be worn by the patient during radiographic examination (Figs 7.1A to E).

The purpose of diagnostic radiographic templates is to incorporate the patient's proposed treatment plan into radiographic examination. Following are requirements for radiographic diagnostic templates.

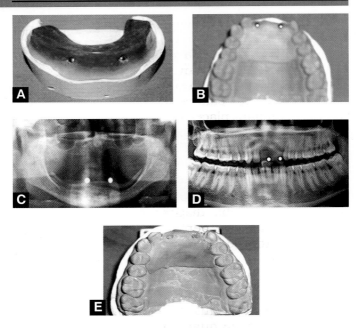

Figs 7.1A to E: Diagnostic stents for recording panoramic radiograph (A) For completely edentulous patient (B) For dentulous patient. Panaromic radiograph with steel spheres at the proposed implant sites (C) For completely edentulous patient (D) For dentulous patient (E) Diagnostic stent converted into surgical stent by removing the steel spheres

1. Mounted diagnostic casts.
2. Diagnostic wax-up.
3. It is copied in clear acrylic.
4. Radiopaque material, barium sulphate, gutta-percha or ball bearing inserts are placed at selected areas and radiographs are taken in mouth.
5. CT or OPG are taken with template in mouth.

Surgical Template

Usually radiographic templates are converted into surgical template; which helps to decide probable implant location and angulation. The diagnostic stent was converted into surgical stent by making a hollow space over planned implant site. This stent helped in implant placement at exact location so as to ensure the restoration of esthetics, speech and function.

Radiographic Assessment of Implant Cases

Preoperative radiographic assessment remains one of the most valuable diagnostic tools to develop a surgical plan from perspective of function and esthetic restoration.

Objectives of Preoperative Imaging

- To identify disease
- Determine bone quality
- Determine bone quantity
- Determine implant position
- Determine implant orientation.

Various imaging modalities are available such as

Computed Tomography (CT) Scan

Computed Tomography (CT) scans give a very accurate view of anatomical structures. Direct measurements can be made from it. It will be done to evaluate jawbone at the future implant site. Serial axial and coronal sections should be made with slice thickness of 3.0 mm. Bone available in vertical, mesiodistal and labiolingual directions were measured by inbuilt distance cursor present in the

CT machine. Exact position of adjacent vital structures such as inferior alveolar canal, floor of the nasal cavity, floor of the maxillary sinus can be assessed. After the determination of the amount of available bone (length, width and height) and density, surgery for the placement of implants should be planned. The radiation dose to the patients is relatively high so there must be clinical justification for all scans. Introduced in 1970s; it was used for treatment planning in implant dentistry in late 1980s. For the first time, CT made it possible to evaluate anatomy in axial plane. CT is capable of producing 1.5 mm thick cross-section in few minutes only. It can evaluate density of bone in Hounsfield Units (Figs 7.2A to C).

Limitations

- CT produces oblique section
- Metal causes artifacts; so metallic restorations severely compromise the dimensional accuracy of image
- Radiation exposure many times higher than conventional radiography.

Computer-Guided Technology (CAD/CAM)

Surgical planning software and computer-guided implantology allows for the interactive use of CT data combines the 3-dimensional accuracy of CT imaging with computer-aided-design. It enables precise pre-operative assessment. If an appropriate radiographic orientation device has been used at the time of scanning, surgical guides can be constructed by CAD/CAM technology. This allows the operator to

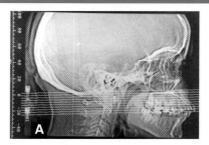

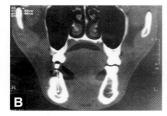
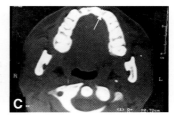

Figs 7.2A to C: Preoperative radiographic evaluation using computed tomographic scan (A) Scout of patient showing divisions of axial scan (B) Axial scan of a patient with the radiopaque marker for measuring the height of bone in the right mandibular first molar region (C) Coronal scan of the patient for measuring the bone width available in the future implant site (Maxillary anterior region)

plan the case, place virtual implants and then construct a surgical guide to aid implants placement.

Tomograms

Tomograms also provide 3-dimensional information and cross-sectional views but are limited to short sections of the mandible and maxilla. Tomograms tend to be less accurate than CT scans and may be distorted-in particular if positioning is not optimal. The main use of tomograms is to provide cross-sectional views of limited anatomical sections for example, in inferior alveolar canal localization and in the assessment of lingual concavities. The main advantage of tomograms over CT scans is the reliance on less expensive equipment. However, when large areas are to be investigated and multiple tomogram section required, CT scans are preferable as exposure to ionizing radiation is reduced. Conventional tomography produces cross sections perpendicular to alveolar ridge and direct measurements can be made from tomogram (Fig. 7.3).

Limitations

- Image blurring
- Lack of cross referring with standard lateral, frontal and panoramic radiographs
- Time consuming if large number of tomograms are required.

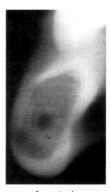

Fig. 7.3: Spiral tomogram of posterior mandible showing inferior dental canal and cortical bone

Orthopantomagram (OPG)

OPG is used to observe the single image of maxilla and mandible in frontal plane. It gives an excellent overall view of the jaws and teeth and is usually the first radiograph taken as part of an implant assessment. As panoramic images suffer limitations of accuracy, further radiographs may be indicated. Diagnostic stents with metal spheres can be placed intraorally during OPG examination.

Advantages

- Single image of maxilla and mandible in frontal plane
- Vertical height of bone initially can be assessed
- Relatively low dose of exposure.

Limitations

- Non-uniform magnification, distortion and overlapping images
- Different parts of radiograph have varying degree of magnification with no single corrective factor being applicable.

To overcome the limitation of the OPG such as non-uniform magnification, distortion, etc. the following formula helps in calculating the true amount of clinically available vertical bone at the planned implant site.

Actual height of available bone =

$$\frac{\text{Radiographic height of available bone} \times \text{Actual diameter of steel sphere}}{\text{Radiographic diameter of steel sphere}}$$

These diagnostic stents can be used both in dentulous and edentulous patients; for exact calculation of bone height. Bone width should be calculated with the help of study models.

Intraoral Periapical Radiograph (IOPA)

Intraoral periapical Radiographs provides detailed information regarding the dimensions in length and height of available bone in small sections. These are most commonly used being inexpensive and of easy availability. These help to rule out any disease at planned implant site. These also serve as part of post-implantation follow up of implant cases for assessment of crestal bone level changes and to detect presence of radiolucent zones around implants. IOPA radiographs can be used in extremely poor patients and immediate implant placement in extraction sites after verification of important anatomical landmarks such as inferior alveolar canal and floor of maxillary sinus. Periapical radiograph provides image of limited region of the mandibular or maxillary alveolus.

Advantages

- Rules out local bone or dental disease
- Common radiograph for postoperative follow up, of implant cases, assessment of crestal bone level changes and detect presence of radiolucent zones around implant
- Inexpensive and easily available.

Limitations

- Distortion and magnification of image

- Limited value in determining bone density or mineralization
- Limited use in depicting the spatial relationship between the structures and proposed implant site.

It is advisable to use a combination of radiographic view to reduce the chance of error. The combination of an OPG and periapical radiographs may be advisable for certain implant procedures.

Occlusal Radiograph

Rarely indicated in implant dentistry because of following reasons:
- Degree of mineralization of trabecular bone is not determined
- Spatial relationship between critical structure such as mandibular canal, mental foramen and implant site is lost.

Lateral Cephalogram

Lateral cephalogram was suggested to be used as a section of mid saggital region of maxilla and mandible.
- It provides vertical height, width and angulation of bone at midline
- Helps to evaluate loss of vertical dimension, skeletal arch inter-relationship, anterior crown-implant ratio, anterior tooth position in prosthesis, etc.

Limitations

- It does not provide an image of exact region anticipated for implant location

- Magnification error was found to be between 6 to 15 percent.

Magnetic Resonance Imaging (MRI)

It is a quantitatively accurate technique with exact tomographic sections and no distortion. It is used as secondary imaging technique when CT fails. It has no radiation exposure.

Limitations

- It is not useful to see bone mineralization, nor a high-yield technique for identifying bone or dental disease
- Expensive and limited availability.

Treatment Planning

Once the decision to provide an implant-supported has been taken, the case must be planned in detail. All options must be considered and presented to the patient, together with details of the advantages, disadvantages, risks, costs and anticipated success. It is felt by some that implants should be last resort and teeth should be maintained at all costs. The high success rate of implant therapy questions this opinion. An essential part of the planning stage is to ensure that environment in which the prosthesis is to be placed as favorable and stable as possible. Treatment planning for the placement and restoration of osseointegrated implants involves the considerations of many variables; including systemic and local host factors and design of prosthesis.

The role of clinician in treatment planning is:
1. To determine if the patient's symptoms would benefit from implant treatment.
2. To decide provisionally what method of retention to the fixtures should be employed.
3. To estimate likely tooth positions.
4. To assess likely occlusal possibilities.
5. To counsel the patient.
6. To make surgical guides and radiographic templates.

Using the study casts and a diagnostic wax-up of the proposed restorations, it is possible to predict the final outcome before starting treatment. A careful note should be made of the following.

- *Proposed occlusal scheme:* It requires for posterior stability and controlled anterior guidance. The aim of posterior stability to distribute axial loading among a reasonable number of posterior teeth. The aim of controlled anterior guidance is to distribute non axial loading away from prosthesis wherever possible. By this arrangement excess load will be avoid to implants. Remaining teeth should therefore be adjusted and restored, as indicated clinically, to create the occlusal scheme most favorable to the long term success of the implants supported prosthesis. When an implant-supported prosthesis is placed, allowance must be made for the physiological movement of remaining teeth and the implant being, in effect, ankylosed. This usually means keeping implant prosthesis and teeth separate

- *The prognosis of teeth* that are key to success to must be assessed carefully by clinical and radiographic means. Where the prognosis is suspect, steps should be taken to limit long term uncertainties. For example, it may be appropriate to place cast restorations on "key teeth" that have a significant risk of fracture

- *Contingency plans for the possible loss of "key teeth"* need to be formulated and recorded before starting treatment. If the loss of a key tooth would seriously jeopardize the success of the treatment, and the prognosis of that key tooth is poor, its removal and replacement should become part of the treatment plan.

EXTRACTION OF TEETH

It is a difficult decision to extract or not the teeth for proper placement of implant and prognosis of implants. The final judgement of extraction of any teeth especially for better placement of implants should be decided by many factors such as

- Prognosis and strategic importance of remaining tooth/teeth
- Outcome of implant prosthesis-whether leaving the tooth will endanger adjacent implants or it may jeopardize the case and reduces the chance of extensive correction
- Tooth/teeth become detrimental to the overall treatment goal, and complicate the treatment process
- Tooth/teeth influence the site of implants
- Prognosis of implants justifies the sacrifice of teeth/tooth.

Timing of Extractions

When a tooth is to be extracted and replaced with an implant, it is necessary to decide whether this should happen immediately or following a period of healing before the placement of the implant. Generally the soft tissue healing occur in one month and bone healing is in excess of four months. The benefits and problems related to these alternative approaches are as follow.

Immediate Implant Placement into Extraction Site

The ideal implant site would be defined as one where there is no hard or soft tissue loss with prosthetic emergence profile identical to a natural tooth. The only site that would come close to this definition is the immediate extraction site. The concept of immediate implantation with root analog implant design and a custom healing abutment is important factor to preserve hard and soft tissue leading to an optimal esthetic result. Immediate post extraction implantation can be predictably performed only in cases where there is no active infection. In cases of active endodontic/periodontal infections the procedure is delayed/staged to 4-6 weeks after extraction.

Advantages

- It reduces time between removal of teeth and restoring the implant
- It preserves bone and soft tissue.

Disadvantages

- Immediate placement may limit the possibility of surgically modifying the soft tissue, as it is sometimes necessary to achieve good esthetics
- It may be difficult to decide on the depth to which to place the head of implant, as hard and soft tissue remodeling varies as the site heals. This may result in either the implant being placed deeper than is ideal, or in exposure of an implant that has been placed too superficially. Multiple units placed in esthetic areas are particularly vulnerable to these variations
- Although it is relatively easy process but some times it needs more expertise and become difficult procedures.

Delayed Placement

Advantages

- Initial remodeling of soft tissue and hard tissue has occurred. This allows for predictable placement of implants in relation to these tissues
- There is more soft tissue available to modify gingival esthetics.

Disadvantages

- Increases treatment time
- If the bone ridge is just wide enough for implant placement at the time of extraction then further resorption may occur if placement is delayed, making subsequent implant placement difficult without tissue augmentation.

The Number and Position of Implants

During formulating a treatment plan involving implants, it is essential to be aware of the dimensions required for implant placement.

- A minimum of 5 mm is required in terms of interocclusal space
- The minimum mesiodistal space for the placement of a single tooth implant is approximately 6-7 mm
- For the replacement of some lower incisors and other such situations thin, narrow implants exits. The strength of such implants, however may be cause of concern.

Planned number and positioning of implant is determined by proposed restoration as:

- The quantity and quality of the bone
- Loads to which restoration will be subjected.

Full Maxillary Fixed Bridge

Typically 6 implants may be used possibly more when available bone is not ideal, or occlusal loads are expected to be more. Implants should be placed at regular interval and correspond to the correct tooth position for the proposed restoration. Limited cantilevers may be considered.

Full Mandibular Fixed Bridge

Bone quality in the mandible is normally better than that found in the maxilla, so fewer implant is required than in the maxilla. Implants are typically placed anterior to the mental foramina and if required distal to the foramina, but clear of the inferior alveolar canal.

Partial Bridge

If three or more units or to be restored, and assuming that the units are to be linked, it is desirable to distribute loads by arranging the implants in a tripod relationship to each other. If this is achieved it is not necessary to place one implant for each missing tooth.

Maxillary Overdentures

These are typically supported by four implants. Various attachments, including bars and studs may be used assuming good separation between implants.

Mandibular Overdentures

Two implants are usually required to retain a mandibular overdenture. If bar is to be used the implants should be placed anteriorly so that a straight bar can be provided. This has the additional advantage of bar not encroaching on the lingual space.

With all overdentures it is essential to have adequate interocclusal space for the attachments. Implants may need to be placed deeper into the bone to obtain the space required. Failure to provide adequate space results in overcontoured prosthesis and thin acrylic, which is may be prone to fracture.

SUMMARY

• Medical and dental contraindications must be fully considered before implant placement and thorough clinical assessment should be made

- Implants are placed in suitable sites in appropriate patients. All treatment option must be considered
- The most suitable radiographic procedures must be selected to give required diagnostic and treatment options. This has to take into account an up-to-date evaluation of comparative radiation dose
- Careful treatment planning using all available technique, including study casts and mocks-up of the final result, is required for a predictable clinical outcome it should be properly done
- A risk assessment is made of various treatment options taking into account the prognosis of all remaining teeth. Extraction of compromised teeth should be done to control these risk factors.

CHAPTER
8

Surgery

INTRODUCTION

The main purpose of implant surgery is to establish anchorage for an implant so that a prosthetics may be most effectively secured in position. In some circumstances, surgical and restorative procedures will be carried out by the same operator, while in others a team of surgeon and prosthodontist will provide the overall clinical treatment. In either situation careful planning of overall treatment is essential if optimum result is obtained. To carry out successful implant surgery thorough knowledge of surgical anatomy and clear view of planned prosthetic outcome is required.

Mandible

Main anatomical consideration when placing implants in the mandible include the:

Inferior Alveolar Canal

The location of inferior alveolar (dental) canal can be a major limiting factor for placement of implant in posterior mandible, as it may influence length of used implant. A clearance of at least 2 mm from the top of the inferior dental nerve should be allowed for the possibility of any surgical trauma. Location of canal is essential for determination of optimal length of implant to be placed (Fig. 8.1). High quality radiographs are a necessary part of the preoperative assessment, and supplementary views may be required during the surgical procedure. Surgical exposure and identification of the mental foramen may be helpful in confirming the position of the canal (Fig. 8.2).

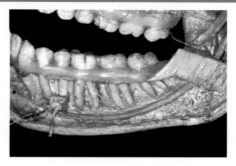

Fig. 8.1: Relationship of teeth with inferior alveolar (dental) nerve

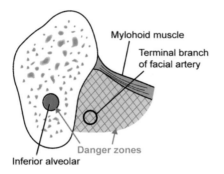

Fig. 8.2: Cross-section view of posterior mandible

Mental Foramina

The inferior dental canal anteriorly opens on mandible through the mental foramina. Anterior to the mental foramina, it is usually possible to place longer implant, given the amount of bone present. If, however implants are to be placed close the foramina, care must be taken to leave a section of the inferior dental nerve anterior to the foramina. The incisive branch of the inferior alveolar nerve which runs anterior to the mental foramina may be damaged by implants being placed in the anterior mandible. Patient may occasionally comments on some altered sensation in the area. This is usually transient.

Submandibular Fossa

The submandibular fossa is lingually positioned to the body of the mandible below the mylohyoid line. The fossa may limit the placement of implants, mainly in posterior section of the mandible. The anatomical shape of the mandible in the region of the fossa varies considerably and in posterior region may take the form of a thin lingual shelf through which penetration may accidentally take place during surgical procedure or implant placement. The position of mylohyoid line can usually be palpated with ease. Sometimes it is necessary to obtain a 3D scan of the area to define the exact shape of the mandible in the region. Facial artery loops over the submandibular gland in the region of the first permanent molar and gives off a substantial terminal branch in the form of submental artery. This is at risk of damage in the anterior aspect of the fossa, possibly as for forward as the canine position.

MAXILLA

Maxillary Sinus

The maxillary antrum is often a major limiting factor for the use of implants in the posterior maxilla,

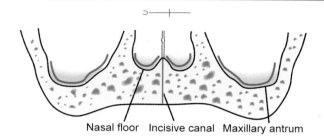

Nasal floor   Incisive canal   Maxillary antrum

Fig. 8.3: Surgical anatomy of maxilla showing sites where implant
placement may be restricted

frequently making implant impossible without
resorting to the bone augmentation procedures. It
should be noted that if planning to extract maxillary
premolar and molar teeth before implant placement,
the removal of teeth may initiate pneumatization
of the antrum into the alveolar process. This results
in a reduction in the bone available for implant
placement (Fig. 8.3).

Incisive Canal

The neurovascular bundle contained within the
incisive canal is positioned in the midline, palatal
to the central incisor teeth. If implants encroach
on this canal, soft tissue rather than hard tissue
union can be expected in this area. Depending on
the extent to which an implant encroaches on the
incisive canal involvement of this anatomical
structure may adversely influence the success of
the implant placement.

Bone Quality

Bone quality is important in implant success. Typically, the ideal bone is of good vascularity with an adequate cortex and medullary bone of reasonable density. The anterior mandible is considered is good site and posterior maxilla which may have thin cortex and sparse medullary space is generally considered to be least favourable site implant placement. Bone quality has been classified into four types. Type IV bone is worst possible bone environment for implant placement because of inadequate stability and poor bone quality.

Surgical Technique

The procedures is carried out after careful planning and involves precise soft tissue handling and bone preparation. To minimize thermal injury to the bone technique requires intermittent drilling technique, copious irrigation, fresh drop drills, and controlled cutting speeds. It should be carried under sterile conditions.

Implant Positioning

The position of implants is dictated by the intended position of the final restoration, not solely by the availability of bone. It is one of the major problems regarding failures of implants. Following guidelines are essentials in preoperative treatment planning for surgical phase of treatment.

Radiographs

Presurgical radiographs must be used to assess availability of bone. The use of tomograms, CT scans, axial tomograms (OPG), periapical radiographs will be helpful to decide implant placement.

Study Casts

Articulated study casts are very valuable in assessing tooth position, angulation and key features of edentulous spaces. Measurement can be made and proposed restoration and implant position is defined. A diagnostic wax up on the cast of the proposed restoration can be great value and will allow the precise construction of a surgical guide. It is important to remember that study casts show soft tissue shape rather than hard tissue shape; this may be very misleading. The relationship between bone and soft tissue can be assessed with the aid of radiographs. However, sounding the bone and transferring the information to a sectioned cast is a helpful adjunct (Fig. 8.4).

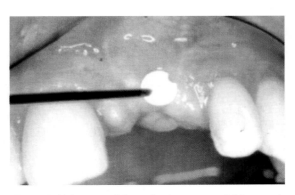

Fig. 8.4: Using a straight probe to measure thickness of soft tissue—'ridge mapping'

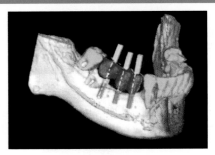

Fig. 8.5: CT scan of the mandible using interactive 3D planning and simulated surgery

Surgical Planning Software

The interactive use of CT data allows for the virtual placement of implants in precise relationship to the proposed final restoration. The software may be used to construct computer generated surgical guides (Fig. 8.5).

PROCEDURE OF IMPLANT SURGERY IN DENTAL CLINIC

Placement and restoration of implants are usually performed in stages. The first stage involves the surgical part where the actual implant is placed into the bone. The implant is left alone for period of 4-6 months depending on the bone quality and allowed to heal and to become osseointegrated. A second surgery is required in which the implant is uncovered and exposed through the oral environment with a healing cap placed to ensure proper healing of soft tissue around the site of the future abutment. Restorative phase then follows with the placement of abutments, either a fixed partial denture or a removable denture (overdenture).

There are some implant systems that require only one surgical intervention, and implant is immediately placed in contact with the oral environment.

Preoperative Documentations

a. *Dental Investigations*
   - Study models
   - OPG
   - Intraoral periapical X-rays
   - Presurgical prosthetic mock-up
   - Surgical stents [CT scan, etc.].
b. *General Investigations*
   - Biochemical analysis
   - Systemic medical problems
   - Habits evaluation.

Presurgical Treatment

During presurgical treatment planning, oral health and hygiene of patients should be improved. This initial therapy besides scaling included restoration, endodontic treatment, prosthetic rehabilitation, etc. for full mouth before implant surgery.

Premedication

Patients should be premedicated with suitable antibiotics, anti-anxiety drugs from the previous day of proposed surgery. It may be oral or intravenous. Patients will be also advised to use chlorhexidine mouth wash 2-3 times daily, 3 days prior to surgery.

OT Preparations Included

- Scrubbing dental chair and unit with bactericidal solution

- Carbonization of floor
- Fumigation of the operating room with formalin will be done a day prior to surgery
- All operative instruments, drills, drapes should be autoclaved
- Sterilized implants should be used
- Disposable pre-sterilized syringes, needles, gloves, Bard-parker blades No. 15, 11 black non-absorbable 3-0 silk sutures, etc. should be used.

Preparation of the Patient

- Ensure that the patient fully understand the surgical treatment
- Confirm that informed consent for the procedure has been given and is documented
- Provide the patient with a head cover and protective glasses
- Apply sterile draping with a complete or upper body drape
- The surgeon should now scrub and grown-up
- Ensure that there is good illumination of the operative site.

Basic Instrumentation

- Surgical drapes
- Surgical hoses
- Dental explorer
- Scalpel
- Needle holders for suture material
- Various retractors
- Gauge.

Surgical Armamentarium Used for Implant Placement (Figs 8.6A to D)

A saline coolant must be delivered during surgical drill.

Principal of Incision Design

The site, size and form of the incision should be planned to give the best possible access and ensure the least damage to important structures. This will

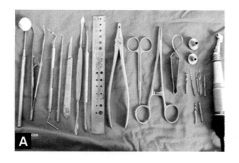

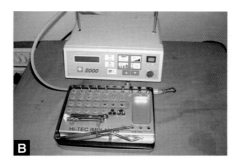

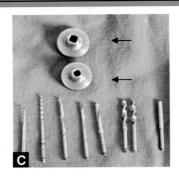

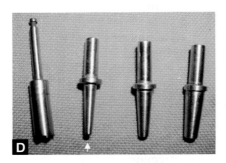

Figs 8.6A to D: (A, B) Physiodispensor, torque control hand piece and other surgical instruments (C) Finger keys, round bur and surgical drills (D) Tissue punch and condensers of gradually increasing sizes

also ensure good wound closure, minimize the risk of any possible nerve damage, and aid the visualization of defects, concavities and perforations.

Flap reflection is usually best done with a periosteal elevator or Mitchell's trimmer, to avoid the tearing the flap.

An incision should:

- Provide good access and visibility of the operative site
- Provide flexibility in positioning the surgical guide
- Allow identification of important anatomical landmarks, e.g. the mental foramina and incisal canal
- Facilitate the identification of contours of the adjacent teeth, and concavities or protrusions on the surface of the bone
- Have clean edges, which will facilitate primary closure and optimize healing by primary intention
- Permit the raising of a full mucoperiosteal flap, ensuring that it has a good vascular supply
- Minimize scarring and avoid vestibular flattening.

Maxilla

Crestal Incision

This may be with or without a relieving incision. A relieving incision will:

- Provide the surgeon with increased visibility. This particularly important when concavities are present on the buccal aspect of the ridge
- Allow for good access for the surgical stent
- Result in less scarring
- Avoid vestibular reduction as a result of scar formation.

Vestibular Incision

This incision was previously the standard procedures for two stage implant placement, ensuring that the implant was completely covered and protected during the healing phase. It is also claimed to provide a superior vascular supply, and there would be no contamination of implant from the oral environment (Incision site distant to implant). Disadvantages of this technique were that it caused vestibular flattening and increased scarring. Vestibular flattening made it difficult to insert the denture after implant placement, unless extensive reduction of buccal flanges of the denture was carried out. Failure to reduce these sufficiently resulted in the wound being open.

Comparative studies between crestal and vestibular incisions have shown little difference in the outcome of both incisions.

Mandible

Crestal Incision

This gives the same advantages as in the maxilla. A careful blunt dissection is required to identify the mental neurovascular bundle, and it is important to expose the mental foramina to identify any anterior loop. Tissue separation with a blunt instrument will show if the inferior alveolar nerve is approaching the mental foramina from a distal or a mesial direction, and should confirm what is already visible on radiographs. The use of metal instruments when reflecting the mucoperiosteal flap near the mental foramina should be avoided; reflection is better carried out with a damp piece of gauze.

Drilling Equipment

Most implant systems provide a drilling unit with variable speed and torque settings, however drilling units are available that are not device specific.

The osteotomy site generally prepared at 1500-2000 rpm to prevent overheating. Following preparation of the site, the insertion of the implant and/or tapping of the site are carried out at about 25 rpm and torque limit of up to 40 N cm, depending on bone density.

FIRST STAGE SURGERY

The proposed surgical site will be anesthesized by infiltration of 2 percent lignocaine with 1:100000 epinephrine. After anesthesia is effective, stent will be placed in the mouth; point of entry should be marked deep in the bone through the guiding hole made in the stent using a sharp straight probe. Incision parallel to the mid-crestal line, slightly lingual was made using B.P. knife and buccal mucoperiostal flap is raised. After raising the flap on the surface of bone, point of entry is seen as bleeding point. One can also simply take out a round piece of tissue with help of tissue punch which should be slightly bigger that implant size. Reflection of flap deprives the bone from periosteal blood supply. Drilling must be started at marked point in the predecided direction.

Since bone is susceptible to heat, drilling efforts must be made to control the temperature during the process of drilling and maintain the temperature below 47°C to prevent bone necrosis. Drilling is done at low speed of 800 to 2000 rpm, without applying pressure. Drilling should be intermittent and a pause of 5 seconds is given after every 5 seconds of drilling to avoid overheating of bone. During the process of drilling copious irrigation should be done throughout the procedure with cool sterile saline solution. Initial bone preparation to desired depth will be done with pilot drill (diameter 1.25 mm) keeping the angulation checked in buccal lingual and mesiodistal directions. The graduated twist drills (diameters 2 mm, 2.2 mm, 2.8 mm and 3 mm) should be consecutively used, to enlarge the diameter of the osteotomy and maintaining the same orientation of drills. The angulation as well as the depth of drilling will be checked continuously. Drilling is done gently in straight, deliberate, precise up and down motion with low pressure, low speed. Copious irrigation must be done to avoid overheating and necrosis of the alveolar bone.

The implant is then placed into the osteotomy preparation, the finger key is engaged to the head of implant, and the implant will tightly screwed into bone with gentle pressure till the neck of the implant is in alignment with crest of bone. Depending on different types of implant there is some time osteotomy preparation is needed before insertion of the implant. The implant should be never forced with excessive pressure to avoid micro-cracking of the bone. The flap is repositioned and sutured carefully with 3-0 black non-absorbable silk suture, without creating any undue pressure on the suture line. Accurate repositioning and suturing contribute considerably to fast and undisturbed wound healing and integration of the implant.

As a general recommendation, whenever possible implant should be inserted in such way that they engage two cortical plates to facilitate better primary anchorage of the implant. This is normally achieved by engaging the plates in the coronal and apical regions: however buccal and lingual plates can also be used. This is particularly the case when working above the inferior dental nerve, where engagement of the inferior border of the mandible could be very hazardous (Figs 8.7A to I).

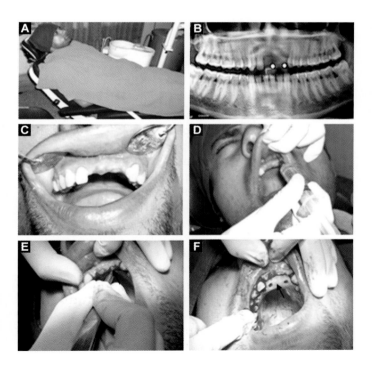

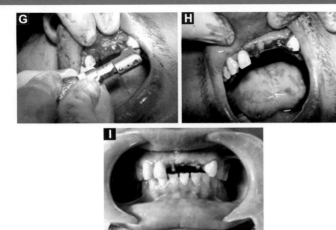

Figs 8.7A to I: Various steps involved in the process of single piece implant placement in single stage surgery (A) Patient in implant clinic (B) Panoramic radiograph with steel spheres at proposed implant sites (C) Intraoral pre-implantation view (D) Infiltration of anesthetic (E) Incision parallel and slightly lingual to midcrestal line (F) Surgical stent in place (G) Osteotomy preparation using drills (H) Implants after surgical fixation (I) Implants after healing

In the maxilla it is often possible to establish bicortical stability using the sinus or nasal floor. Only the apical tip of the implant should engage the cortical plate.

Manufactures supply various drilling systems with facility to provide irrigation to operative site (Fig. 8.8).

After completion of suturing, a bolus of moist gauze (pressure pack) is applied over surgical site for compression. This helps in homeostasis thereby reducing the possibility of formation of hematoma.

Patient was advised to follow post-surgical regime which included:

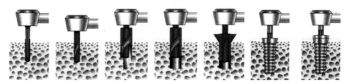

Fig. 8.8: Figure showing drilling sequence using different drills and placement of implant as well as final cover screw

- Removal of pressure pack after one hour
- Not to spit or rinse vigorously
- Cold packs for 8 hours
- Not to smoke, drink or use tobacco in any form
- Not to touch sutures and wounds
- Soft nutritious diet for 3-4 days
- Maintain oral hygiene.

Patient should be called after 24 hours for post-operative check-up. Sutures will be removed after 7 days. IOPA X-ray was taken to examine the initial level of bone.

Abutment Selection

While abutments may be selected at time of implant insertion, which can have logistic advantages, this better done after second stage surgery, either in laboratory using a cast prepared from a fixture head impression or by direct measurement at chair side.

Single or Two-stage Surgery

If it is intended to bury the implant during healing period, a short cover screw or healing abutment is attached. This approach necessitates a second surgical procedure. If second surgical procedure is to be avoided then along healing abutment that protrudes through the soft tissue is fitted. This single stage procedure is not indicated in all situation, in particular, if there is risk of denture pressing integrating implant or, if the implant is short or located in less than ideal bone. If long healing abutment is placed the soft tissue must be carefully adapted around it.

SECOND STAGE SURGERY

The aim of second stage surgery is to uncover the implants and place healing abutments, which will:
- Facilitate gingival healing
- Allow easy access to the implants following healing.

Second stage surgery is required to uncover a buried implant following osteointegration. This may be done using a tissue punch or more typically by raising a mucoperiosteal flap. Healing abutment designed to protrude through the soft tissues are attached to the implants during this period.

Surgical Procedures

Edentulous maxilla; placement of four implants for retaining an overdenture:

- Crestal second premolar to second premolar. This is necessary to enable dissection to expose the incisive foramen. A buccal relieving incision is often needed to expose any buccal concavities.

Implant placement:

- Canine and central incisor regions. Where there is lack of bone in the incisor region then implant may sometimes be placed in the premolar regions.

Suggested prosthesis:
*   Bar retained complete overdenture.

Edentulous maxilla; placement of six implants to retain a fixed prosthesis:

Suggested incision:
*   Crestal first molar to first molar, necessary to dissect to expose incisal foramen. Buccal relieving incision to expose any buccal concavities.

Implant placement:
*   Depending on floor of maxillary sinus, and bone volume in second premolar, canine and incisor regions.

Suggested prosthesis:
*   Fixed, with cantilever extension approximately one and half times the distance between the most anterior and distal implants, up to a maximum of 15 mm, depending on the lengths of the implants and bone quality.

Edentulous mandible; placement of two implants to retain an overdenture:

Suggested incision:
*   Crestal first premolar to first premolar, not necessary to dissect down to expose mental foramina.

Implant placement:
*   Canine region approximately 2 cm apart. Where the form of edentulous ridge is curved, then it may not be possible to link the implants rigidly without encroaching on the lingual space. In these circumstances it is usually necessary to use individual ball attachments.

Suggested abutments:
• Either ball or bar retained prosthesis.

Edentulous mandible; placement of five implants to retain a fixed prosthesis:

Suggested incision:
• Crestal first molar to first molar relieving incision anteriorly, if necessary blunt dissection to expose both mental foramina.

Implant placement:
• Suggested locations 3 mm in front of mental foramina, minimum distance between implants 7 mm (centre to centre) following the curve of anterior mandible, with access through, or slightly lingual to, the cingulam of the lower teeth.

Suggested prosthesis:
• Fixed with cantilever extension approximately twice the distance between the most anterior and distal implants, up to maximum of 15 mm from the distal aspect of the abutment.

Posterior Mandible

Suggested incision:
• Crestal, with relieving incision anteriorly to mental foramina and blunt dissection to expose these as necessary.

Implant placement:
• Suggesting spacing 3 mm distal to the natural abutment directly medial to the edentulous region. Optimum separation between implants 7 mm (center to center) using surgical guide.

Posterior Maxilla

Suggested incision:
• Crestal with relieving incision anteriorly.

Implant placement:
- Suggested 3 mm distal to the direct medial abutment. Optimum separation between implants 7 mm using surgical guide.

Single tooth:
- *Suggested incision:* Crestal with relieving incision if necessary.

Immediate Placement

It refers to placement of implant into extraction site immediately following removal of the teeth/tooth (Figs 8.9A to E).

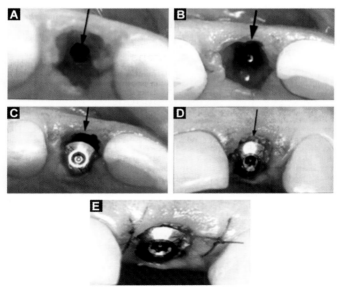

Figs 8.9A to E: (A) Tooth has been extracted (B) Osteotomy has been prepared in palatel aspect of extraction socket (C) Implant has been inserted (D) Graft material is placed between mucosal tissue and abutment, (E) Tissue sutured

- As the implants is unlikely to fit extraction socket perfectly especially if the implant is cylindrical design, it usually necessary to extend the implants apical to the socket to provide this fixation. Immediate implants should be placed in molar sites with extreme precaution because the inferior dental canal or maxillary sinus and root shape of molar teeth tends to make the socket shape unsuitable for immediate implant placement
- As the buccal aspect of many tooth roots tends to be covered by very thin bone, great care must be taken during extraction to keep the bony socket intact
- The ideal position for implant is rarely the same as the position of the root socket
- Care should be taken for proper axial position and proper placement in bony socket to avoid unfavourably positioned and inappropriately exposed.
  - Osteotomes should be used to minimize the trauma associated with extraction.
  - Following extraction of tooth, careful debridement of the extraction socket should be carried out to remove any remnants of tissue.
  - It is preferable to engage bone on the palatal aspect of the socket (to avoid the risk to penetrate buccal concavity).
  - Following the insertion of implant, it is often preferable to follow a single stage surgical protocol and place a healing abutment.
  - In suturing the socket, primary closure of the soft tissue wound should not be attempted.

Immediate Loading

It may be possible to restore implants immediately upon placement, however, in certain situations this may lead to an increased risk of failure. This method may be considered in specific cases, such as the anterior mandible, which normally has a good quantity and quality of bone. Use in single tooth case may also be considered, however it is extremely important to avoid any functional loading of the temporary crown in all mandibular movements.

Reasons for Failed Integration

- Poor surgical site
- Inexperienced operator
- Failure to achieve primary stability
- Early loading
- Poor surgical technique
- Infection
- Heavy tobacco—smoking habit.

SUMMARY

Insertion of implant—a surgical template is fabricated, which is used as a guide during drilling (Figs 8.10A and B).

Following steps are carried out in the insertion phase of two stage implant

A. *Incision*—for one tooth replacement small crestal incision is given, and minimal flap retraction is done. For full arch implant surgery incision can be designed as the situation demands.

B. *Osteotomy preparation (drilling)*—drilling can be either sequential (starting from the smallest drill and gradually increasing drill diameter and

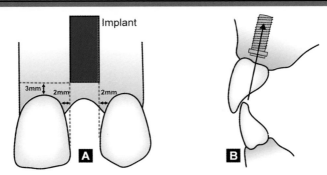

Figs 8.10A and B: (A) Typical relationships and distances between adjacent teeth and implants. (B) Opposing tooth position is a very good guide to implant position (the long axis of implant should approximate with the incisal edge of the lower incisor)

usually up to 0.25 mm less than the implant diameter or only using the same diameter drill as the diameter of the implant (press fit implant).

Drilling is done intermittently to avoid necrosis, speed should be 800-1000 rpm and the torque 30-45 ncm, (threshold temperature for osteocytes is 43-47 degree centigrade). Preferably copious internal irrigation should be done.

C. *Insertion of screw*—after osteotomy completion implant is inserted and tightened with the help of wrench. Paralleling pins are used if another implant is inserted in the vicinity of the first implant to maintain the parallelism between the two implants.

D. *Cover screw*—in two stages implant system inserted screw is covered by a cap, made up of metal or plastic, known as the cover screw or healing cap.

E. *Suturing*—suturing is done with catgut or silk (interrupted mattress sutures are preferred). The cover screw is either left open in the oral cavity or submerged in the flap.

After 3-4 months, at second stage surgery the implant site is re-opened and the cover screw is taken out. Gingival former is fitted on the implant screw for one week.

In one stage implants, cover screw and gingival former are not required, as we directly go for prosthetic work just after the insertion of the implant in the bone.

Keys to Successful Surgical Placement of Implants

- A precise knowledge of surgical anatomy is required before implants placement
- A careful technique during preparation of bone is essential to avoid overheating and subsequent damage to the bone
- The use of surgical guide is often recommended for exact positioning of implant
- Careful manipulation of the soft tissues is required for a good aesthetic result
- Placement of implants immediately into extraction socket is successful procedure (except molar teeth) if implants can be rigidly fixed into bone.

CHAPTER
9

Prosthodontic Procedure: Single Tooth Implant

INTRODUCTION

Before implant surgery is contemplated the team must have agreed with the patient on detail treatment objectives. Implant treatment must be based on a comprehensive history, through clinical examination, careful diagnosis and agreed treatment plan. Effective and close teamwork is therefore, essential between those providing the surgery and those responsible for the construction of prosthesis, which of course, includes the dental technician.

Prosthodontic procedure related to implants is similar to other conventional crown and bridge procedures in many ways. The ease of restoration depends on the position of the implant. Ideal implant placement is sometimes difficult to achieve, and a functional or aesthetic compromise usually ensues (Figs 9.1A to C). Vast majority of implants treatments provide satisfactory functional and aesthetic results. If we are critical of the outcome of implant treatments, the main criticism would relate to the preservation and management of soft tissues, namely the interdental papillae. Sometimes when multiple implants are placed there is some reduction of the papillae, referred to as "blunting".

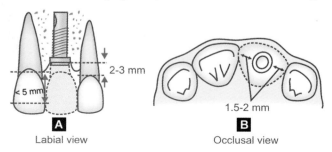

Labial view | Occlusal view

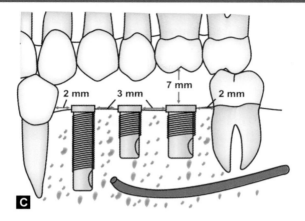

Figs 9.1A to C: Ideal placement of single implant and multiple posterior implants

RESTORATION OF SINGLE TOOTH IMPLANTS

When aesthetics are important, notably in anterior part of mouth healing period should be allowed to the gingival tissues to take up a stable position. Implant should be aligned in such way that the long axis is in line with incisal edges of the adjacent teeth.

When providing posterior restorations, the healing time is not so critical. Some recession of gingival margin may, however be anticipated when prosthodontic procedures are started within 3-4 weeks of time for posterior crowns, the long axis of the implant should be aligned so that the screw access comes through the central fossa of the premolar or molar tooth.

Minimum requirements for the single tooth implant

- Standard implants—3.75 mm diameter: Ideally suited for replacement of upper central incisors, upper and lower canines and upper and lower premolars
- Narrow implants—3.3 mm diameter: This implant is well suited for replacement of upper lateral incisors and lower incisors
- Wide implants—5 or 5.5 mm diameter: This diameter is ideally suited for replacement of single molar teeth.

Basic principles related to implant placement for single teeth as follows:

- Use the longest implant that is possible without interfering with key anatomical structures
- Have an implant length to crown height ratio of greater than one
- Loads are best directed down the long axis of the implants and should be aligned with the overlying crowns
- Single implants should not be used to support cantilevers.

PROSTHETIC STAGES OF TREATMENT WITH SINGLE TOOTH IMPLANTS

Timing of Prosthetic Treatment

It is better to leave the healing abutments in place until the gingival tissue around them has matured.

Type of Restoration

There are two types of restoration:

- A screw retained prosthesis secured direct to the implant

- A cement retained prosthesis secured direct to an abutment.

Abutment Selection

The role of abutment is to connect the final prosthesis to the implant body. Most manufacturers provide a range of designs; however, these are usually product specific. These abutments are following three types:

Manufactured Precision Abutments (Machined abutments)

Material of Manufacture

- Titanium

Advantages

- Simple to use
- Minimal chair side and laboratory time
- Predictable fit with implant prosthesis components
- Good retention.

Prepable Abutment

Material of Manufacture

- Titanium
- Gold alloy
- Ceramic.

Advantages

- Suitable for all cases
- Allows for angulation changes
- Modification allows for good gingival contour.

Disadvantages

*   Increases clinical and laboratory time

Customized Abutments

Material of Manufacture

*   Gold alloy
*   Titanium
*   Zirconium
*   Ceramic.

Advantages

*   Suitable for all cases
*   Allow for angulation changes
*   Modification allows for good gingival contour.

Disadvantages

*   Increases clinical and laboratory time
*   Material choice influenced by occlusal loads.

SEQUENCE OF EVENTS FOR TREATMENT WITH A SINGLE TOOTH MACHINED ABUTMENT

*   Removal of healing abutments and placement of machined abutment
*   Radiographic confirmation of abutment placement
*   Tightening of abutment screw with a torque wrench
*   Impression procedures using an impression coping
*   Jaw registration
*   Shade taking
*   Temporization
*   Try-in and cementation or screw retention.

It is generally recommended that wherever, it possible, it is better to leave the healing abutments in place until the gingival tissue around them has matured. A minimum of approximately 4 weeks from the time of second stage surgery is recommended. Where the implant has been inserted with a surgical phase sufficient time should pass to allow the gingival tissue to mature. If there is poor positioning of the implant, the use of a customized abutment may be appropriate.

It is important to follow the manufacturer's protocol and guidelines for each abutment system.

Impression Procedure

Most implant systems provide a premachined impression coping for recording an impression of the head of implant. This is usually made up of two pieces: the impression coping and guide pin. With a machined abutment it is necessary to use a preformed plastic or metal impression coping (Figs 9.2A to D).

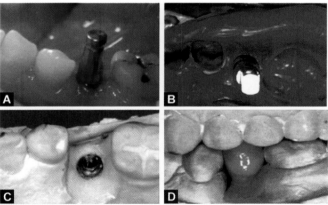

Figs 9.2A to D: (A) Intraoral view of transfer impression coping in place (B) Transfer impression-analogue assembly placed into elastormeric impression (C) Cast of implant analogue with soft tissue cast removed (D) Completed restoration in occlusion and working casts

A polyvinyl silicone or polyether impression material may be used. Following complete setting of the impression material the tray is removed from the mouth. Impression coping is incorporated within the impression. Careful inspection of the impression will confirm stability of the impression coping and accurate recording of the relevant hard and soft tissues. Impression should be washed and disinfected before being dispatched to the dental laboratory.

Occlusal Registration

The maxillary cast should be mounted in a semi adjustable articulator with a face-bow transfer.

If a sufficient number of occluding teeth are present, the cast may be mounted in the intercuspal position without the aid of a wax jaw registration.

In replacing an anterior tooth there should be light occlusal contacts in the intercuspal position, while in protrusive movements these should be smooth and similar to those on remaining anterior teeth.

If the intercuspal position is not precise or there are multiple missing teeth, then the use of an occlusal rim or jaw registration with acrylic bonnets will help facilitate the mounting the casts. It is recommended that wherever possible a mutually protected occlusion should be provided. That is scheme in which there are stable occlusal contacts in the posterior part of mouth in intercuspal position (ICP), and where possible no working or nonworking contacts on the implant retained prosthesis. Canine guidance, if present on the natural teeth, should be provided on the implant stabilized prosthesis.

Shade Taking

Shade taking and completion of the laboratory prescription is same as other fixed prosthodontic procedure. All ceramic crowns may be preferred in anterior teeth according to there indication but most of time porcelain fused to metal crown is preferred due to its durability and occlusal or incisal guidance and occlusal forces.

Prescription should be send to laboratory with specification whether a metal framework or ceramic coping is required.

Temporization

Temporization at the end of the impression procedures usually takes the form of protective silicone cap. If temporary tooth replacement has been provided in the form of a partial denture or a resin bonded bridge, these restoration needs to be adjusted to fit the new abutment surface. Alternatively, a temporary crown or bridge may be made at this stage, using techniques similar to those used in conventional bridgework. Advantage of using temporary crowns or bridges are that appearance and function can be assessed before making a definitive restoration. The soft tissues can also be supported and to an extent moulded to improve contours.

Customized Abutments

The indication for use of customized abutment is in those types of cases where dental implants have been placed inappropriately, for facilitation of prosthodontic procedures. With some implant systems angulated abutments are able to overcome certain problems. It is more common, however for customized abutments to be produced in the laboratory. Impression procedures differ slightly in that fixture-head impression is required.

Impression coping is attached directly to the implant fixture head.

An open tray technique is required whereby the impression coping can protrude through an opening in the impression tray. After impression has been taken the impression coping is unscrewed to allow withdrawal of the impression from the mouth. Some implant system include a push-fit attachment for impression coping. In the laboratory fixture head - working cast is produced. This allows a customized abutment is produced, reangulating the retaining core to favorable position. Such customized abutment can be made of gold alloy, titanium or ceramic. It is good practice to make a temporary crown at this stage. Once the abutment is placed, further working impression is required. Success rate of cemented crowns appears to be good. Initially there were concerns as to whether cemented crowns and abutments would loosen and there would be some need to employ a retrievable system. Alternatively single crowns can be made a screw retained crowns, which incorporate the abutment attach directly on to the implant, avoiding the need for intermediate abutments. Such crown may on occasion be more bulky than cemented crowns but preferred by some clinicians.

CAD/CAM-derived Abutments

This is relatively new development is likely to assume increasing importance as manufactures develop the technique. These abutments have advantage that the design is carried out using specialist software. It has disadvantage that at present it has no three dimensional orientation with the opposing or adjacent teeth. It is possible to make abutments in titanium or a ceramic, which is considered to be more biocompatible material.

Fitting the Completed Restoration

On the day of fitting the completed restoration, the temporary prosthesis should be removed. The new crowns may then be seated with finger pressure. The contact points are checked with dental floss as for conventional crowns.

Occlusal contacts should be checked prior to cementation and should follow the occlusal pattern on the master cast. There should be light contacts as the patient goes gently into intercuspal position. The crowns should be checked for lateral, working, nonworking and protrusive movements.

Cementation with temporary cement may be prudent when placing the final restoration. This will give time for the soft tissues to adapt, while simplifying removal and modification of implant crown if required. In cases where abutments have been used the abutments screws should be tightened to manufacture's recommended values before the final cementation.

Following cementation an IOPA radiograph is taken to:

- Verify the seating of the restoration
- Check for excess cement
- Record a base line marginal bone height
- Prosthesis should be reviewed after regular interval

Danger signs at review appointment:

- Cement failure
- Loosening of abutment screws
- Fracture of veneering material, ceramic or resin
- Fracture of abutment screws
- Increased bone loss around an implant
- Fracture of implant.

If any of above has occurred a careful diagnosis should be made of the cause. Repeated failure to diagnosis the problem will lead ultimately to failure of prosthesis or implant.

The most common causes of these problems are:

- Occlusal overload; careful review of all occlusal contacts in all patterns of mandibular movement and their refinement may be needed
- Failure to use a nocturnal occlusal guard especially in patients having evidence of parafunctional activity
- Faulty construction
- Off-axis loading of an implant.

SUMMARY

Fabrication of prosthesis—following steps are performed in this stage:

A. Attach the impression post on the implant in patient's mouth.
B. Make impression of the implant with the post attached in patient's mouth.
C. Remove the post from the implant, and fix this post in the impression in the inverted manner and fix the implant analog on this post.
D. Now, pour the impression with the impression post and analog assembly.
E. Analog will be in the cast.
F. Remove the impression post from the analog.
G. Fix the abutment on the analog.
H. Fabricate crown on this abutment (on the cast).
I. Fix the abutment on the implant in patient mouth.

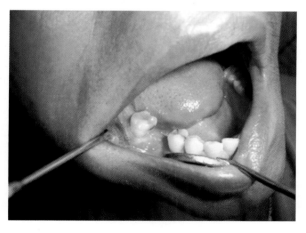

Fig. 9.3: Pre-op photograph

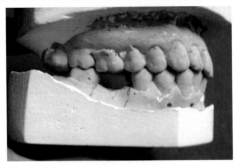

Fig. 9.4: Diagnostic casts

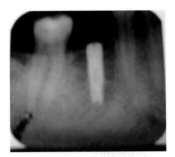

Fig. 9.5: Radiograph (immediate post-op)

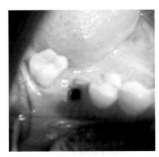

Fig. 9.6: Removed cover screw (after 2nd stage surgery)

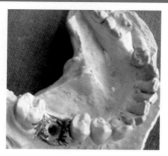

Fig. 9.7: Analog in the cast

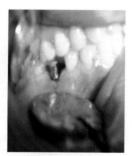

Fig. 9.8: Abutment is fixed on the implant

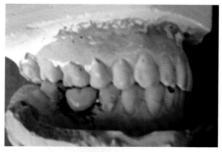

Fig. 9.9: Crown fabricated

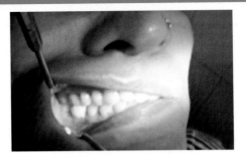

Fig. 9.10: Crown cemented

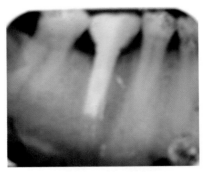

Fig. 9.11: Post-op radiograph 6 months after loading

J. Fix the crown on the abutment either by cement or a screw, after establishing proper occlusion (Figs 9.3 to 9.11, single tooth implant case).

CHAPTER 10

Prosthodontic Procedure: Partial Replacement Case

The provision of dental implants for the partially dentate patients may be preferred option where:

- Certain key teeth have been extracted from the arch;
- A traditional dental bridge abutment has failed and cannot be replaced by another natural tooth;
- A localized fixed structure would reduce the coverage of a removable partial denture.

Methods for Replacement for Edentulous Spaces in the Arch

- Observation
- Removable partial denture
- Adhesive bridgework (Resin retained bridges)
- Conventional bridgework
- Implant stabilized prosthesis.

All remaining teeth should be assessed for their restorative, endodontic and periodontal status. A decision on their individual prognosis may influence the overall plan and decisions regarding planning for future implants.

Where implant treatment is contemplated the diagnostic casts may be used for:

- A general occlusal examination over the full range of mandibular movements and their effects on an implant retained prosthesis
- Diagnostic wax-up or tooth set-up
- Construction of a radiographic stent
- Sectioned casts in conjunction with ridge mapping
- Construction of a surgical stent.

Radiographic Stent/Template

Various forms of radiographic templates have been described using acrylic stents incorporating metal markers, coated with metal foil or made from a radio-opaque resin. The ideal form should be one which, in combination with a suitable radiograph such as a spiral or computed tomography (CT) will show ideal final tooth position and its relationship to remaining bone.

Surgical Stent

A surgical stent that fit correctly on natural teeth adjacent to the edentulous space is an essential aid to position the implants.

Mechanical Consideration for Implant Placement

- Longer implants are to be preferred to shorter ones, provided that excessive heat is not generated during their insertion
- Bicortical fixation is to be preferred
- Implant placement in denser, but not highly dense, bone is to be preferred
- High occlusal loads indicate the use of more implants. History and examination can provide information related to this, e.g. tooth wear, a history of bruxism or tooth clenching, bulky masticatory muscles and fractured restorations or teeth
- Loads are best directed down the long axis of implants
- Cantilevers should normally be shorter than the separation of the closest two implants.

- Implants should not be angulated towards each other to the extent where restoration is precluded.

Aesthetic Considerations
- Implants should be in alignment with the overlying crowns
- Implants should not be closure than 3 mm, where they are parallel
- Implants and their projected connecting components should be contained within the prosthetic envelope
- Implants and their projected connecting components should not prevent oral hygiene.

In partial replacement cases, prosthodontic procedures are very similar to those for restoring a single tooth implant. As the span increases there are more indications for additional prosthodontic procedures to ascertain accuracy of fit and jaw registration. Procedures tend to be as follows:
- Abutment selection
- Radiographic confirmation of abutment fit and use of torque wrench
- Impression procedures
- Verification of accuracy of working cast
- Jaw registration
- Tooth try-in
- Metal try-in
- Try-in of final restoration placement.

In certain circumstances some of these stages can be undertaken during same appointment. Temporization at this stage may be patient continuing to wear partial dentures, a temporary conventional bridge or resin-bonded bridge. This may be made at the chair side, but tends to be more durable if made in the laboratory. The use of such temporary bridges can allow the clinician to assess the initial aesthetics, the occlusion and soft tissue response to the proposed long-term restoration. In partial replacement cases, it is usual to provide a fixed bridge restoration. Occasionally, if implant abutment are limited, or there has been failure during surgical stage, the use of removable partial overdenture may be considered as an interim or rescue prosthesis.

Abutment Selection for Fixed Partial Prosthesis

Pre-machined Manufactured Titanium Abutments
- Simple to use
- Minimal chair side and laboratory time
- Predictable fit.

Customized Abutments
- Gold/titanium/ceramic
- Suitable for all cases
- Can allow for angulation changes
- Modifications promote good gingival contours
- Increase in clinical and laboratory time needed.

Impression Procedures

Impression procedures for dental implants usually make use of manufactured impression transfer copings. These are designed to fit on either the implant body, sometimes called fixture head copings (impression procedures are known as fixture head impressions) or the implant abutment, sometimes called abutment copings (impression procedures are known as abutment impressions). The copings may remain in the impression when it is removed, being secured to the implant or abutment with a screw so that they may be disengaged before the impression is removed. These are often called pick-up copings and the impression is called a pick-up impression. When abutments have been individually prepared, then impression procedures similar to those used in conventional fixed prosthodontic techniques may be employed (Figs 10.1A to E).

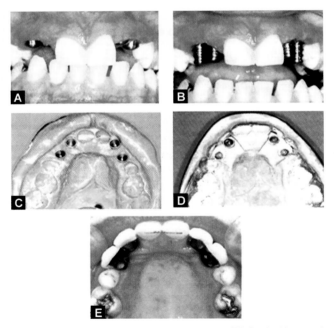

Figs 10.1A to E: (A) Healing abutments in place (B) Conical impression copings in place (C) Working impression (D) Working cast with surgical template in place (E) Splinted crowns in place

Primary Impressions

Following second stage surgery primary impression may be recorded by an alginate impression material. After primary cast can be constructed and special tray may be made.

Special tray may be constructed with an open window where the impression copings are to remain in impression or in a closed design if they are to be reseated in the impression after its removal from the mouth.

Selection of Impression Material

An elastomeric impression material polyether or polyvinylsiloxane impression materials should be used for better accuracy.

Impression Recorded at the Level of the Top of the Implant

It should be done for following reasons:
- To decide the type and size of abutments in laboratory after construction of a master cast
- To provide a master impression for constructing one piece prosthesis designed to fit directly on the implants
- To construct a master cast for the use of prepable abutments or custom-made abutments.

Abutments-level Impressions

Impressions may be recorded following abutment selection and placement. Measurement from the head of the implant to the margin of mucosal cuff will aid in determining the height of necessary abutments to be used.

Occlusal Registration

It is recommended that the casts for all partially dentate cases should be mounted on a semi-adjustable articulator. This will require appropriate occlusal records and a face-bow transfer for mounting the maxillary cast. Where there is an insufficient number of occluding teeth to permit freehand location, then records suitable for mounting the casts in the intercuspal position (ICP) will be needed. A fluid interocclusal recording material is placed between the opposing teeth to get desired jaw relationship.

Temporary Prostheses

It may be help in aesthetics or phonetics and function. This may be adjusted clinically by addition and removal of material to provide the optimum contours, and can help in achieving the optimum shape for prosthesis before making final version. Such temporary prosthesis are frequently made using manufactured polymeric components. Some patterns of which can be placed directly on the head of implant. It is recommended that these should be screw retained, since this permits repeated removal and replacement, which can facilitate incremental modification. This can be valuable where it is desired to gradually modify the contours of adjacent soft tissues. If the prosthesis is made of acrylic resin it is frequently necessary to incorporate a strengthening device.

Occlusion

The design of occlusion in the partial dentate case requires careful consideration. As we know that the physiologic mobility of natural teeth is absent in the implant, we should avoids transfer of excessive forces to the implants by adjustment of occlusion.

To minimize lateral loads on posterior implant prosthesis, disclusion should occur in lateral and protrusive movements. This may not be possible when a natural canine is to be replaced with prosthesis; however it is recommended that there should be shallow disclusion, and group function should be avoided.

Posterior implant-stabilized prosthesis where a canine is not to be replaced, the occlusion should be arranged to provide:

- Contact of opposing natural teeth
- Multiple light contacts in intercuspal position
- No working or non working interferences.

When canine is to be presents, the occlusion should be arranged to provide:

- Multiple light contacts in intercuspal position,
- Opposing natural teeth,
- Shallow canine disclusion,
- No working or non working interferences.

For anterior bridgework in these situations the occlusion should be arranged where possible to provide,

- Multiple light contacts in intercuspal position,
- Shallow anterior disclusion shared by the prosthetic teeth.

Choice of Materials

The occlusal surface for the prosthesis may be made of:

- Porcelain
- Acrylic resin

- Composite resin
- Metal.

Choice of Materials are Depends by Following Factors

Space Restrictions

Limited interocclusal space between the head of implant and the opposing arch may require the use of a metallic occlusal surface.

Number of Implants in the Construction

In a large reconstruction using more than four implants, the use of a polymeric material would make repair and maintenance simpler instead of prosthesis having porcelain veneer.

Amount of Hard and Soft Tissue to be Replaced by Prosthesis

A large, bulky prosthesis replacing both hard and soft tissue become difficult to fabricate using porcelain, veneering with modified acrylic resin is to be preferred.

Evidence of Parafunctional Activity

A more resilient material such as acrylic resin may be preferred.

Insertion of Prosthesis

In many cases, the patient has significant hard and soft tissue loss. If patient is not willing to consider tissue grafting, the use of acrylic flange or pink porcelain on a porcelain-fused to metal super-structure can produce an acceptable result.

Complexity of the prosthodontic phase treatment increases with the number of implants. If screw retained restorations is planned, the ideal positioning of dental implants allows the screw access to be lingual to the labial face of the replacement teeth. This is less critical if a cemented

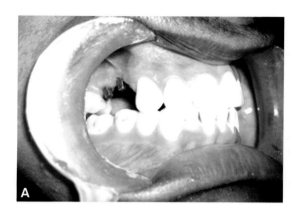

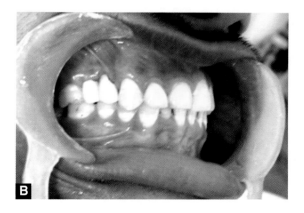

Radiographic Follow Up

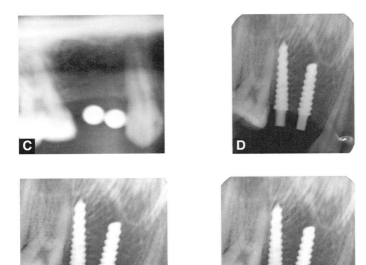

Figs 10.2A to F: (A) Implants placed in 14, 15 region (B) Implant supported temporary crowns (C) Pre-implantation radiograph (D) 3 months post-implantation (E) 1-year post-implantation (F) 1.5 years post-implantation

bridge is planned, in a particular if it involved the use of customized abutment. If the implant is placed deeply, it is possible to use machined angulated abutments to reposition the screw access channels into a more favorable position (Figs 10.2A to F Case Report).

CHAPTER
11

Prosthodontic Procedure: Edentulous Case

Restoration of one or both edentulous jaws with prosthesis stabilized by dental implants is appropriate in two situations.

- First and more commonly, when a conventional complete denture is found to be unsuccessful.
- Second situation, is the desirability of promoting the retention of alveolar bone and avoiding resorption and future atrophy of edentulous jaw.

In the restoration of complete dental arch by means of implants, two options are available to the practitioner, namely:

1. Fixed-implant retained prosthesis.
2. Implant-supported overdenture.

FIXED-IMPLANT RETAINED PROSTHESIS

Followings factors are determining factor to decide complete implant-stabilized fixed prosthesis(es) as influencing factors;

- Number of implants: Adequate quality/volume of bone for minimum 5-6 implants in the maxilla and 4 implants in the mandible
- Total retention and stability of prosthesis
- Reduced volume/mucosal coverage improving tolerance
- Optimal masticatory function
- Where resorption has created inadequate height and width to the jaw, autogenous grafting may be used in the form of an inlay or onlay
- Cantilevering limits occlusal table
- Risks destabilizing an opposing complete denture,
- More difficult to clean and achieve good oral hygiene.

- Presence of periodontally compromised natural teeth may compromise implant support
- Initials casts greater than overdenture.

A fixed prosthesis may be choosen to oppose an intact or partially dentate arch of natural teeth. If entire length of the occlusion is to be restored either sufficient bone must exist above the maxillary antrum or inferior dental canal to accommodate implants at least 6-7 mm length and 5-6 mm diameter. If not, then an auxillary surgical procedure must be considered, e.g. a maxillary sinus lift, in order to create an increased volume of bone. A fixed mandibular prosthesis occupying a reduced prosthetic space may be provided to oppose a complete maxillary denture, if upper foundation offers good support and retention. As for occlusion is concerned, loads should be spread widely, avoiding local high concentration. Optimizes the number and position of implants with heavy loads, provide biteguards for night wear. Canine guidance should be avoided. Modified acrylic resin material for artificial teeth or composite veneering most commonly used (porcelain teeth may be used for overdentures).

IMPLANT-SUPPORTED OVERDENTURE

This procedure is mainly determined by the number of implants present and need for flange. Following are influencing factors (Figs 11.1A and B):
- Number of Implants for overdenture in maxilla-4 implants and mandible-2 implants
- Enhanced stability and retention by anchorage from implants in a resorbed jaw

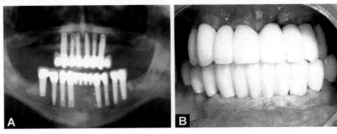

Figs 11.1A and B: (A) OPG view of implant supported denture
(B) Artificial denture on implants

- Improved resistance permitting improved tooth positions in the dental arch
- Facial support provided by denture flange
- Occlusal table may oppose an intact natural arch
- Complete denture occlusion favors stability of an opposing denture having limited support from the jaw
- Easy cleaning for oral hygiene
- Higher maintenance requirements.

Completed dentures may be successfully stabilized by a limited number of implants sited in the edentulous jaw. A sufficient volume of bone for implantation is usually present in the canine eminence and anterior to antrum in the maxilla and canine/first premolar area of mandible (although the central incisor site may also be available). Generally, standard implants of approximately 4 mm diameter and at least 10 mm length are considered adequate to sustain load in the maxilla, whereas even 7 mm is a sufficient length to engage the more dense basal bone of the anterior mandible. The longer the implant, the better are the prospects for osseointegration and the reaction to loading. Essential features for planning an implant-supported complete denture are to be maintained. Occlusion relation against natural arch should to avoid canine guidance, and against complete denture should be balanced occlusion.

Prosthodontic stages for a full arch restoration is as follows:

- Primary impression for special tray
- Secondary impression with an open-tray technique and impression copings
- Verification of the cast if multiple implants are used
- Jaw registration, which is most likely to require an occlusal rim
- Wax try-in
- Metal try-in for framework
- Wax and metal try-in or metal/porcelain try-in
- Finish.

With a complete arch restoration much of the planning of tooth position equates to the standard prosthetic techniques for complete dentures. Assessment of the occlusal vertical dimension, occlusal plane, tooth position, centerline, smile line and retruded contact position (RCP) are all important to the success of the case.

Abutment Selection for Complete Fixed-Implant Prosthesis

Premachined

Standard abutments:
- Appropriate for oil rig design, typically in mandible

- Aesthetics not significant
- Minimum of 4 mm spacing between each one
- Easy to clean.

Wide platform abutments:
- Meet criteria for standard abutments
- Enhance loading potential in molar areas of jaws.

Multi-unit abutments:
- Alternative to standard abutment
- Appropriate for optimal emergence profile from good ridges forms, e.g. maxilla.
- Facilitate sitting of cylinder component in the 'prosthetic envelope'.

Angulated abutment:
- Necessary where long axis of implant body and tooth crown are divergent, e.g. Class II div 2 incisor pattern
- Compensate for differences in implant/ posterior arch alignment
- Avoid perforating buccal/labial tooth face with a channel for access to the prosthesis screw.

Customized

Individually fabricated by casting onto a gold alloy abutment post, milling a precision abutment (clinic/ laboratory)/CAD/CAM produced by scanning, milling/spark erosion of a titanium block.
- Optimize emergence profile of the unit
- Optimize superstructure form in relation to the restored arch.

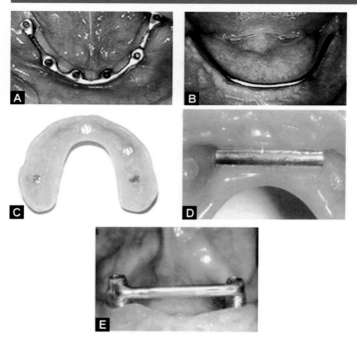

Figs 11.2A to E: Different attachment of overdenture

Overdenture can be retained in the following ways (Figs 11.2A to E):
• Bar and clip
• Ball attachment
• Magnets.

Tissue bar constructed for removable prosthesis, sometimes attachment can be placed distal to last attachment.

A bar and clip design is the most popular, as it gives the patient confidence with minimal maintenance. Ball attachments are simple and allow the patient to clean effectively. It is suggested that the ball abutments be used in the mandible and not in the maxilla. Magnets have certain advantages, but are less commonly used, as they are bulky in design and may corrode in clinical service (Figs 11.3A to H - Case report).

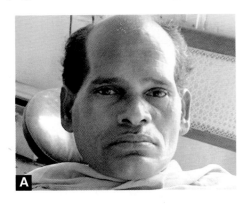

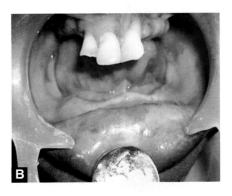

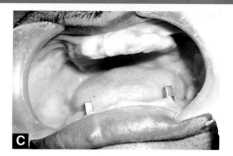

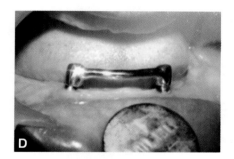

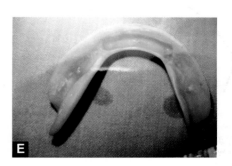

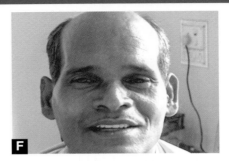

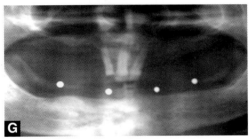

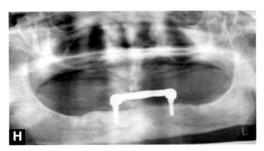

Figs 11.3A to H: (A) Pre-implantation extraoral view (B) Pre-implantation intraoral view showing atrophic mandibular ridge (C) Implant placed in premental region (D) Cast metal bar placed over implants (E) Mandibular denture maximally extended to reduce stresses over implants (F) Patient wearing implant supported overdenture (G) Pre-implantation panaromic radiograph (H) Post-implantation panaromic radiograph

In case of overdenture, abutment is attached to the denture base by certain attachments. In ball and ring type of attachment ball like head of the implant is protruded in the oral cavity (male part) and inserted into a socket housing on the tissue surface of denture, called "o" ring (female part). In a bar attachment bar is fabricated on 2 or 4 implants inserted in the jaw and a clip is housed in the tissue surface of the denture, which fits on this bar which ultimately improves retention and stability of the denture.

LABORATORY CONSIDERATIONS

The clinician's responsibility is to provide work of the highest possible quality. This should be mirrored in the dental laboratory with accurate and skilled manipulation of materials. Communications and good relationship between clinicians and dental technicians reduce the chance of errors. Ultimately, the responsibility for the finished prosthesis lies with the clinicians.

Laboratory stages will be familiar to most readers as:

- Production of working cast
- Selection of component and design
- Wax-up to full contour
- Casting of metal superstructure
- Veneering with porcelain, acrylic or composite.

Dental materials are constantly evolving to enhance clinical performance and appearance. All porcelain restorations have been introduced for single tooth restorations. A strengthened core is cast or milled to fit the fixture head or implant abutment.

Surface abutment is then fired to produce the desired contour and shade.

CAD/CAM

Computer aided design/computer aided manufacture (CAD/CAM) has recently been developed for use in implantology. Various procedures have been employed utilizing laser scanning, sparked erosion and milling techniques. In this way a single abutment or frameworks can be produced.

SUMMARY (PARTIAL AND COMPLETE PROSTHESIS)

Healing period of 4-6 months is allowed before loading the implant with final restoration. Progressive loading should be given by initial placement of transitional prosthesis of acrylic material, with no occlusal contact. After rigid fixation of the implant the acrylic transitional prosthesis should be given occlusal contact. Subsequently, it mut be followed by permanent restoration.

The permanent restorations can be made of:
a. Gold/Gold alloys
b. Metal ceramic crown
c. Ni-Cr alloys

Resinous occlusal surfaces are preferred to prevent traumatic shock-type forces from affecting the health and longevity of the osseointegrated interface.

In complete edentulous patient, initially provisional denture should be provided which had been relieved in the regions of the implants for 3 months. Implants loaded, placing resilient material between the implant and the denture. Patient should be recalled for follow-up:

- Ideal surgical implant placement allows the use of standard components and impression procedures
- Fixture level impressions and use of custom abutments, as is standard practice with some implant systems allow restoration of difficult cases
- Cemented implant crowns and superstructures give the best appearance occlusally, whereas screw retained prosthesis allow easier maintenance
- Temporary prostheses give the clinicians and the patient the opportunity to assess the appearance and function prior to completing the laboratory prescription.

Implant Placement in
Advanced Cases and
Other Applications

INTRODUCTION

Good implant therapy results should be expected in those type of cases in which single tooth or a small number of teeth that have been removed atraumatically are to be replaced. The prosthetic management conforms to the existing dentition and supporting tissue.

As the number of teeth to be replaced increases so does the complexity of planning and the method of treatment. More time will be required in more complexes and extensive cases for both the clinical as well as laboratory stages. If the dental arch is edentulous, multiple fixtures will be required. It may be that a number of teeth can be saved. In such cases a decision has to be made as to whether to link the implants to the teeth or to provide a number of independent implant retained units.

Aesthetics

It is simpler to achieve a good aesthetic result if a full arch superstructure is totally implant supported. The most predictable way of achieving a good aesthetic result in such situation is by means of an implant-retained overdenture. There is good opportunity to control the aesthetics at the wax try in stage of treatment. The dental surgeon and technician have full control over the position and arrangement of the teeth, together with the gingival margins and contours of the prosthetic soft tissues. If there have been limited alveolar resorption, there will be problems accommodating the bulk of an overdenture.

When implant-retained fixed bridges are provided, there is less room for adjustment, as the fixture dictates the shape of the superstructure. If there has been minimal alveolar resorption, it can be difficult to create ideal gingival margins, contours and emergence profiles, unless the implants have been placed in an ideal position. With further alveolar resorption, pink porcelain is required to simulate gingival tissues. Some fluting is important to allow effective cleaning of the implants and mucosa.

When teeth and implants are used to support a superstructure, it becomes particularly difficult to provide a continuous gingival margin and uniform emergence profile for the teeth included in the prosthesis. If very few teeth remain and they have dubious prognosis, a case can be made for their removal to simplify implant treatment, improve the aesthetic outcome and enhance long-term success.

Temporary Superstructure

The use of temporary superstructure in full arch cases can be considerable assistance in developing an acceptable aesthetic outcome. As it is difficult to make durable all acrylic temporary superstructure, there period of placement should be limited to a certain periods. If the time required for refining the temporary superstructures needs to be longer than this, it is prudent to consider some form of metal or glass fiber-reinforced temporary superstructure. Such superstructures involved more laboratory work and costs, but sometimes essential.

Impression Procedures

Impression procedures are complicated if prepared teeth and implants are included in a single impression. Often multiple impression procedures are required, involving the use of impression copings. The aim of pick-up impression is to locate dies of teeth and implant analogues within a single master working impression from which a master working cast can be produced. It is good practice, to verify the accuracy of a working cast. This will reduce the risk of errors in fit and occlusion at later stages. Verification bars to link implants abutments can be made on the working cast, which can then be checked in the mouth. These are important measures to avoid errors being compounded during the laboratory phase of treatment.

In the past it was difficult to provide large gold alloy casting of appropriate accuracy for implant superstructures. Casting difficulties are reduced if small units are planned. Various soldering and laser-welding techniques have been developed to join small castings to form large full-arch units, and casting techniques have also improved to accommodate the fine tolerances required. More recently titanium-milled castings have been provided good fit when used with a fixture head impression technique.

Maintenance of a full mouth reconstruction is simplified if small units have been employed. A porcelain fracture in a three units components much easier to deal with than the same fracture in a 12-14 unit full arch reconstruction. Back up dentures or temporary fixed bridges are always useful when the replacement or maintenance of such superstructures is required. It therefore follows that the construction and maintenance of full arch reconstruction, using two fixtures in the mandible and an implant-retained overdentures, is simpler than a full arch fixed bridge supported by 8-10 implants.

Traditional teaching has advocated avoiding the joining of implants and natural teeth. It is known that teeth have some three dimensional physio-logical mobility, but implants have none. It had been thought that joining implants to teeth might result in the early failure of implant screws or the cement lute. Joining implants to teeth can however be successful. A stress broken design using a fixed movable joint has also been employed successfully. Another combination is to use conventional cementation of the retainer on the tooth and screw retention only on the implant. It is not known which arrangement will perform best in the long-term, but clinical experiences indicate that these combina-tions are not as problematic as first thought.

Dental Implants and Periodontal Disease

There are two main problems when considering the placement of dental implants that have or have had periodontal disease:

1. Remaining teeth have poor prognosis.
2. Persistent pathogenic periodontal bacterial flora may adversely affect some dental implants, leading to a loss of osseointegration.

In common with all sound treatment planning, primary dental treatment needs should be met before definitive treatment is carried out. In a patient who has severe periodontal disease, with many teeth having a poor prognosis it is unreasonable to consider implant therapy. It is considered not good to place dental implants in a patient who has advanced uncontrolled periodontal disease. There are however a number of case reports showing the successful placement of dental implants in a patients who have been successfully treated for periodontal disease.

Severe periodontal diseases increase the mobility of natural teeth and are associated with increased recession of the soft tissues and in many cases, drifting of the teeth. Such presenting feature makes it very difficult to achieve a good aesthetic result.

Immediate Implant Placement

All extractions of teeth are accompanied by some alveolar resorption and gingival recession. This is accelerated if a mucosal-born denture is used to replace the lost teeth. Alveolar resorption may be greatly reduced if the tooth roots are retained as overdenture abutments. Similarly, if dental implants are placed into an extraction socket, alveolar resorption may be reduced. Immediate implant replacement is worthy of consideration when single-rooted tooth extraction are planned. Primary stability of the implants can be achieved, if the implant site preparation is deeper and wider than the tooth socket. The use of conical root form implants may be considered an advantage. If the labial alveolar plate is lost during difficult extractions, primary implant stability is difficult to achieve. There are numerous descriptions of using autogenous bone or bone substitutes to fill dead space in extraction socket. The use of such materials may not be necessary if small space exists between the implant and wall of socket. The technique is generally contraindicated if there is any bony pathology, such as a periapical lesion or following a vertical root fracture. It is also difficult to apply the technique in the sites of multirooted tooth extractions. In such situation, it is preferable to allow healing over three to four months before placement of an implant.

Tissue Augmentation

Substantial loss of hard and soft tissue may occur with trauma, periodontal disease and the treatment of neoplastic disease. In patients with hypodontia the alveolar ridges are underdeveloped, given the absence of permanent teeth. In cases in which the tissue loss occurred some months or years previously, a number of techniques may be used to augment the tissues, namely:
• Bone graft
• Soft tissue graft
• Guided tissue regeneration (GTR).

Grafting Material

Important Properties

It should be:
• Sterile,
• Non-toxic

- Non antigenic
- Biocompatible
- Osseoconductive
- Osseoinductive
- Easy to use.

Sources of Autogenous Bone Grafts

Intraoral:
- From the drilling site
- Local to the implant site
- From the mandible anterior to the premolars
- Retromolar region of mandible.

Extraoral:
- From the iliac crest
- From the cranium
- From the radius of maxillomandibular reconstruction.

The gold standard for augmentation technique is the use of the patients own bone.

Common sites for bone grafts are as follows:
- Chin or retromolar area (when small amount of bone is required)
- Hips or ribs (when more extensive bone grafting is required)
- A number of novel techniques have involved harvesting bone from lower leg and the skull.

Scientific research over recent years has been aimed at providing bone substitutes to reduce risk to the patient. In case of sever bone loss corticocancellous bone blocks are required from the hip or ribs to restore whole arches in the form of onlay or inlay bone grafts. These are most commonly placed over maxilla or into the maxillary sinus or nasal apertures. Usually large bone grafts are supplemented by packing particular bone or bone substitutes into the recipient site to create smooth contours. A careful, meticulously planned technique is essential to avoid postoperative complications.

In anterior mandible there is usually sufficient bone to place implants even in the presence of severe resorption. In the posterior mandible inferior alveolar nerve can preclude simple implant placement. It is often preferable to consider nerve repositioning or lateralization of the inferior alveolar nerve in preference to extensive bone grafting in this area. This is often associated with some altered sensation, which can be permanent.

Factors Affecting Prognosis of Bone Grafting
- Asepsis
- Soft tissue closure
- Defect size and topography
- Autogenous bone
- Space maintenance
- Healing time
- Graft immobilization
- Blood vessels-host bone, soft tissue
- Growth factors
- Collagen
- Calcium phosphate.

Layered Approach to Bone Grafting

The host site includes both hard and soft tissue is prepared before the placement of the graft. The bone site is prepared by eliminating any soft tissue on the bone ensuring no infection is present. The soft tissue is prepared by raising the periosteum near the depth of reflection only and attempting to maintain the blood supply from muscles to the periosteum. The soft tissue is expanded to ensure tension free closure.

The autogenous bone is placed directly on the host site and immobilized by fixation and/or tent screws. Blood vessels from the bone must grow into the site rapidly if the portion of the bone graft is to remain vital.

The intermediate layer of the graft, when autogenously bone is not readily available is bone substitutes, which is covered with a barrier membrane. Advantage of the layered approach is that most keys to bone grafting are incorporated.

Soft Tissue Grafting

Connective tissue grafts are able to improve gingival or mucosal contours. Although they do not contribute to bone volume which does not facilitate implant placement if the bone is insufficient. They may however be used as a supplementary measure if severe tissue loss has occurred. A number of periodontal plastic-surgical techniques exist to regenerate lost interdental or interimplant papillae.

Guided Tissue Regeneration (GTR)

Guided tissue regeneration has been used in periodontal treatment for many years. Its use in implantology is more recent. The same principle of bone healing is applies. Epithelial and connective tissues are excluded from the healing site and bone allowed to grow preferentially around the implant. It is important for the membrane to cover the whole defect and to be held rigidly in place. It is common to use particular autogenous bone or bone substitutes as a part of GTR technique to enhance bone healing. Bone tacks are usually used to secure the membrane.

Graft Materials

At present there are four principal categories of material used to augment the bone which will form the floor of the maxillary sinus:

- *Intraoral or extraoral autographs:* Readily available and is the first choice of bone grafting material used to augment the bone for many clinicians.
- *Allografts:* These are graft material derived from the same species, i.e. bone derived from cadavers and have been used widely in orthopedic and periodontal surgery. The graft may be freeze dried or decalcified freeze dried material. It may be harvested from donors with well documented medical histories and is tested for all common antigens during production. It is therefore considered a relatively safe source of grafting material.
- *Xenografts:* Xenografts are made from bovine bone from which the proteins have been removed are purely mineral grafts but have been found to be effective when mixed with the patients blood and packed with sinus.
- *Alloplastic Grafts:* Synthetic alloplastic grafting materials have reduced risk of cross conta-mination and may well act as a good framework for bone formation.

Advantage of Tissue Augmentation
- Facilitate implant and aesthetics.

Disadvantage
- Increase treatment times
- Complexity of treatment
- Cost.

Sinus Lift/Elevation Procedures

The maxillary posterior quadrant poses special challenges to the successful use of implant prostheses. Loss of alveolar ridge, particularly where there has been pneumatization of edentulous posterior maxilla, means that there is frequently a lack of bone height for implant placement (Figs 12.1A and B). This problem can often be managed by surgically augmenting the maxillary sinus floor. In the classic approach, access to the sinus is gained via a bony window created in its buccal wall.

Contraindications

- There must be no sinus pathology
- Patients with acute sinusitis

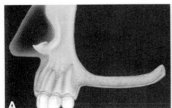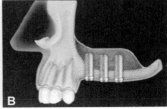

Figs 12.1A and B: (A) Inadequate space for placement of implants in the posterior maxilla (B) Maxillary sinus augmentation for placement of implants

- Tobacco smokers
- Patient with excessive interarch distance.

Procedures

Careful radiographic analysis will indicate the proposed crown to implant ratio of the prosthesis.

It should be carried out under local anesthesia.

Good access is obtained through a wide based soft tissue flap; usually the sinus wall is thin and can be seen as a bluish-grey bony surface.

Using a large rose head burr and copious saline spray, a window can be gently removed in the bone, care being taken not to perforate the underlying sinus membrane.

The inferior and lateral cuts are carried completely through the bone, while superior cut should only perforate the bone. Once the cuts are completed it is possible to move the window upward with gentle pressure. This effect will gradually elevate the sinus membrane, which should be gently lifted of the surrounding bone.

It is important to keep the sinus membrane intact throughout the procedure; perforation is difficult to repair but may sometimes be accomplished with collagen strips. Elevation is continued until the desired size of void has been created.

Other Applications for Osseointegrated Implants

Intraoral:
- Immediate implantation of anterior mandible (teeth in a day)
- Assisting orthodontics

- Rehabilitation of the resected mandible
- Rehabilitation of the resected maxilla.

Intraoral and facial skeleton
- Zygomatic implantation for atrophic maxilla.

Extraoral/facial
- Ear, eye, nose prostheses
- Bone anchored hearing aid (BAHA)
- Linked or stabilized prostheses for maxillofacial rehabilitation.

Immediate Loading

Dentist and patients would like to see the healing times required for the implant treatment reduced to a minimum. It is considered reasonable to load implants in the mandible 3 months after placement and 5-6 months after placement in maxilla. Many patients would like to have 'same day teeth'.

For single tooth or small span bridges it may also be possible to consider immediate loading. Once implants have been surgically placed, appropriate abutments can be placed on the fixtures as long as they have good stabilization. While surgical field is still open, temporary crowns or bridges can be made and cemented or screwed onto the abutments. Thereafter the soft tissue can be replaced with careful suturing technique. It is important that the temporary crown or bridge is relieved partially or totally from occlusion in the intercuspal position and lateral excursions.

Sitting of Dental Implants in Resected Mandible

Partial rim resection or a full-thickness defect of mandible has a major impact upon the masticatory function and quite often the appearance of the patient. Appropriate recovery may demand a bone graft to provide continuity to the jaw, and result will be dependent on the restoring part of the dental arch with a fixed prosthesis stabilized by dental implants. The equivalent result is rarely if ever achieved with conventional denture, which lacks the support, stability and retention provided by dental implants.

- Sufficient good quality bone should be there.
- Allowing emergence of abutments through accessible, immobile soft tissue
- Appropriate to the prosthetic space
- Offering support to the planned arch in occlusion.

Assessment of Resected/Reconstructed Mandible

- Does the jaw articulate satisfactorily with the skull without limited gape, deviation on closing and impaired dental occlusion?
- Do the tongue, lips and cheeks function satisfactorily during deglutition, chewing and speaking?
- Is there access to the site of resection, unimpaired by the tissue contraction/grafts?
- Is there sufficient bone, appropriately aligned with the maxillary/dental arch?

Maxillary Defects

Defects of the facial skeleton can arise as a result of developmental anomalies, surgery or trauma where possible, these are often best managed by surgical correction; however this is not always feasible or capable of providing a satisfactory outcome. In these circumstances, patient may be best helped using a removable obturator.

Development of osseointegrated dental implants and those specifically intended for insertion into the facial skeleton, has made it possible to improve obturator stability dramatically.

Suitable sites are:
- Edentulous ridges
- Zygomatic buttress
- Bony orbital rims
- Dorsal aspect of maxilla where it articulates with pterygoids plates
- Occasionally the palatal processes of the maxilla.

Obturators may be linked to implants using either magnets or precision attachments.

Zygomatic Implants

While original Branemark implant was designed as a tooth analogue to be placed partly or totally within the remnants of the alveolar processes, integration can equally occur in other locations. This potential has been used to help the patients for whom conventional implant is restricted. The zygomatic implant represents one such development and is intended for use in upper jaw, where there is inadequate alveolar bone for placing sufficient dental implants (Fig. 12.2).
- The device is much longer (typically 30-50 mm) than standard design
- Inserted into the zygomatic process of the maxilla through the palatal aspect of the residual alveolar ridge.

Indications

It should not be considered as a first line of treatment when treating the edentulous maxilla or

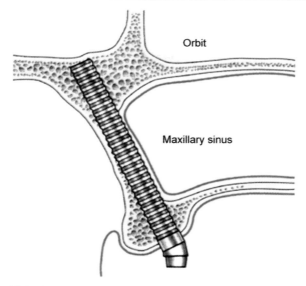

Fig. 12.2: Diagram showing a zygomatic implant engaging the palate and zygomatic bones of the skull lateral to the maxillary sinus and the orbit

one with missing molar teeth, but rather a procedure that may be potentially of value in a small number of cases.

- Can be indicated in edentulous and partially dentate maxillae
- Rarely used on their own, typically combined with other implants/natural teeth
- May enable implantation without bone grafting
- Used with fixed/removable superstructure in the edentulous case
- Can assist in managing the distal extension saddle.

Patient Assessment

- Same basic criteria as for conventional implants
- Special consideration is needed due to potential problems with;
- Access
- Anatomy of surgical site
- Length of implant body
- Location; the head of the implant usually lies palatal to the residual alveolar ridge and is oriented laterally.

Problems

- Same problems as for conventional implants.
- Length, location and orientation pose further potential difficulties.

Facial Prostheses

Facial prostheses that disguise disfigurement resulting from the loss or absence of the eye, nose, ear and lip/cheek can obtain significant stability from specially designed skull implants. In extreme cases, where the defect involves dental, extraoral and facial tissues, a combination of dental and skull implants positioned in accessible bony sites may be used to support and stabilize a combination of prosthesis (e.g. fixed mandibular prosthesis, removable maxillary overdenture or an intraoral and facial prosthesis) (Fig. 12.3).

Treatment Planning for Facial Prosthesis

- Estimation of useful implant sites to provide retention/support for the prosthesis

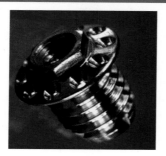

Fig. 12.3: A flanged implant body manufactured for use in the skull

- Consideration of surface contours identifying redundant tissue and penetration by the abutments of unfavorable skin or mucosa
- Determination of the desirable form and border shape of prosthesis.

Radiographic Examination
- CT scan to determine suitable sites for implantation.

Laboratory Assessment
- Download data to analyze the computer image of defect site/selected normal facial tissues
- Construct rapid process model of defect and model of exactly fitting prosthesis
- Construct computer generated template for locating implant sites or
- Produce diagnostic laboratory model for preparation of trial prosthesis
- Prepare preliminary prosthesis, mark implant sites.

Surgical Preparation

- Select likely number, type, position, angulations and relation of implants
- Select one or two stage procedure
- Select likely abutments
  - Penetration of skin ensuring fixed, hair-free site or creating thin grafted site
  - Penetration of mucosa creating thin immobile cuffs within prosthetic space or
  - Replacing skin graft
- Confirm fit of surgical template/mark on facial planes.

Prosthesis Design

- Determine perimeter in relation to fixed or mobile tissue and external form
- Choose retention mechanism, separate or linked abutments using bar, magnets or precision attachment
- Identify space for ventilation
- Consider characteristics (coloration, eyebrows, moustache, hairstyle, spectacles)
- Confirm alignment with normal facial tissues (e.g. eye level, ear prominence).

Bone Anchored Hearing Aids (BAHAs)

Bone anchored hearing aids connected to implants in the mastoid bone of the skull receive direct stimulation and bypass that normally produced in the middle ear. This aid is one alternative to resolve the problems of hearing loss, others being traditional air conducting hearing aids, cochlear implants and surgical procedures such as stapedectomy.

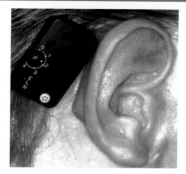

Fig. 12.4: The ear prosthesis and BAHA are slightly separated

Connection to the implant is simply is achieved by the patient inserting the BAHA linkage into a specialized abutment that is screw retained on the top of the skull implant. A single implant is located within the hairline of the patient, sufficiently posterior to the external ear to avoid direct content with helix (Fig. 12.4).

Indications
- Bilateral hearing loss
  - Discharging ears, preventing wearing of air conducting aids.
  - Congenital malformation (atresia) of the outer or middle ear.

Contraindications
- Poor hearing thresholds
- Unilateral otosclerosis
- Mild impairment.

CHAPTER
13

Implants Longevity

There have been several long standing debates about what is considered successful in implant dentistry. It was originally believed that the encapsulation of an implant with a pseudoperiodontium was successful implant until the fixture loosened itself out of the bone. Clinical success is no longer a game of chance. With progress achieved by Branemark in studying osseointegration, a more scientific approach to implant dentistry has emerged.

INTRODUCTION

Several parameters have been suggested in literature for the evaluation of implant's success. The oldest concept being whether the implant is physically retained or removed from the mouth. An implant may be retained in the mouth in situations where prosthetic rehabilitation is not possible, however such implant cannot be considered successful.

Schintmann and Shulman in 1979 suggested that:

- The bone loss up to one third of the height of implant is acceptable
- Dental implant should provide functional service for 5 years at least in 75 percent of cases.

In 1986, Albrektsson et al redefined the success of implants, in terms of mobility, bone resorption, tissue health and retention time. Success rate of 85 percent at the end of 5-year observation period and 80 percent at the end of 10-year period was considered to be the minimum requirement. Interestingly orthopedic implants are less predictable than dental implants with below 75 percent of 10-year survival rate.

Later in 1989, Zarb and Schmitt put four different parameters, for evaluation of long-term effectiveness of osseointegrated dental implants in function, based on the criteria traditionally used in periodontic and prosthodontic clinical evaluation. These measures include:

- Immobile individual implant after removal of prosthesis
- No radiographic evidence of peri-implant radioluscency
- Minimal vertical bone loss around implant as demonstrated by serial periapical radiographs that shows maximum area of bone-implant interface where feasible
- Surgical retrievability of system with minimal morbidity permitting easy resolution of prosthetic problem.

Considering the earlier studies, commonly chosen parameters to assess the implants survival include pain, mobility, gingival health, peri-implant radiolucency and marginal bone loss. These parameters are in accordance with those suggested by Albrektsson et al, Zarb and Schmitt and several others.

PAIN

According to Misch absence of pain under vertical or horizontal forces is the primary criteria for the evaluation of dental implants. Usually, pain does not occur unless the implant is mobile and surrounded by inflamed tissue or has rigid fixation but impinges on a nerve. Tenderness during function or percussion usually implies healing in the proximity of a nerve or bone stressed beyond the physiological limits. Osteotomy preparation and implant placement should be done according to available bone density, height and width to avoid pain.

Pain recorded as occurrence of pain (P/Absence of pain (A) under vertical/horizontal forces/spontaneously.

MOBILITY

Albrektsson, Misch and several others proposed clinical mobility test and stated that implant mobility is a definite evidence of non-integration. Unfortunately, simply the rigid fixation does not guarantee a direct bone-implant interface. According to Misch, a horizontally mobile implant with less than 0.5 mm movement may return to rigid fixation and zero mobility. However, the implants with greater than 1 mm horizontal mobility or any vertical mobility should be removed to avoid continued bone loss.

Implant Mobility (IM) as suggested by Misch recorded as:

- IM0 – Absence of clinical mobility with 500 g in any direction.
- IM1 – Slight detectable horizontal movement
- IM2 – Moderate visible horizontal mobility up to 0.5 mm.
- IM3 – Severe horizontal movement greater than 0.5 mm.
- IM4 – Visible moderate to severe horizontal and any visible vertical movement.

GINGIVAL HEALTH

The marginal peri-implant tissues constitute a functional barrier between the oral environment and the host bone by sealing off the osseous fixture site from noxious agents, and also thermal and mechanical trauma. The ultimate function of soft tissue barrier is reflected in long-term changes of marginal bone height. The inflammation in soft tissue around the implant is more commonly plaque associated however; there could also be acute necrotizing, hormonal, drug induced or spontaneous effects (Figs 13.1A and B).

Quigley and Hein Plaque Index for oral hygiene and Loe and Silness Gingival Index for the assessment of the health of soft tissues around implants are commonly used. The patients are given oral health instructions such as brushing after every meal and use of chlorhexidine mouthwash twice daily for a better prognosis of implant.

Plaque Index
Recorded as suggested by Quigley and Hein

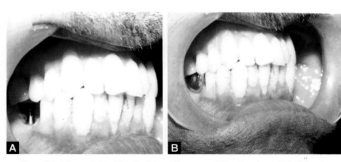

Figs 13.1A and B: Gingival health around the implant (A) Prior to restoration (B) After restoration with gold crown

Grade 0: No plaque
Grade 1: Plaque within apical third of crown
Grade 2: Plaque within middle third of crown
Grade 3: Plaque within coronal third of crown

Gingival Index
Health of the gingiva was assessed as suggested by
Loe and Silness.

Grade 0: No inflammation
Grade 1: Mild inflammation with slight changes in
color and surface; bleeding on probing
Grade 2: Moderate inflammation with redness and
hyperplasia of gingiva, bleeding on probing
Grade 3: Severe inflammation with highly red and
hyperplastic gingiva, tendency to spontane-
ously bleed and ulcerate.

PERI-IMPLANT RADIOLUCENCY (FIG. 13.2)

The union of implant can be through bone as
osseointegration or soft tissue as fibrous union.
Osseointegration is always preferred over fibrous
union of implant. However achievement for
100 percent bony union is not possible and generally
only 60-70 percent of implant surface is in direct
contact of bone. The following could be reasons for
fibrous union.

1. Absence of initial stability of implant.
2. Excessive pressure during implant fixation.
3. Overheating of bone (>47°C).
4. Improper occlusion/parafunctional habits.
5. Improper fitting of the implant in the prepared
osteotomy site.
6. Unsterilized implant having surface impurities.
7. Apical bone necrosis due to overheating.

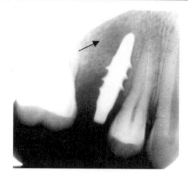

Fig. 13.2: IOPA showing peri-implant radiolucency

Peri-implant Radiolucency: Recorded as: Present (P)/ Absent (A)

MARGINAL BONE LOSS

The level of crestal bone around an endosteal implant should be compared to initial placement position of the implant to find out the marginal bone loss may be primarily attributed to direct surgical invasion and non-infectious tissue reaction immediately after surgery. Amount of marginal bone loss is variable in different cases depending upon the different factors such as initial surgical trauma, infection, improper occlusal contacts and oral hygiene maintenance.

The initial bone loss around the implant is always more than in the following years. Bone loss during the 1st year was approximately 1 mm and after the 1st year the bone loss was 0.1mm/year has been observed by. It should be concluded as an unavoidable change associated with surgical invasion but not always as a result of infection. Exact marginal bone

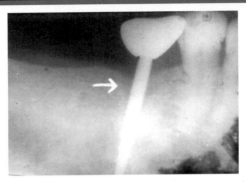

Fig. 13.3: IOPA of a 5-year-old functioning implant-arrow indicates crestal bone loss

loss can not be calculated from radiographs because it is always difficult to obtained complete consistent conditions of radiographs and because of difficulty in 2-dimensional evaluation of 3-dimensional changes. Under ideal conditions a tooth or implant should loose minimum bone. However, it is not possible to determine precisely the extent of bone loss to indicate success or failure of the implant. Some researchers determined that after first year an average of 0.1 mm bone loss was observed in each following year. According to some study bone loss should be less than 0.2 mm annually following the first year of service. A comparative amount of mean bone loss of 0.1 mm to 0.13 mm per year was observed after the first year of prosthesis function by some study (Fig. 13.3).

Presence of peri-implant radiolucency is non-integration, i.e. implant failure. Radiographs demonstrating a seemingly direct contact between bone and implant are considered evidence of osseointegration. Radiolucent zones around the implant are clear indication of implant being anchored by fibrous tissue.

Each implant was assessed by periapical radiographic examination during follow up visits of the patient post-implantation. The level of crestal bone around implant was compared to initial placement position of implant to find out the marginal bone loss.

FACTORS WHICH INFLUENCE IMPLANTS PROGNOSIS

Performing a risk assessment analysis of the patient and minimizing the risk factors involved can maximize clinical survival.

Subject risk includes factors such as cigarette smoking, osteopenia, osteoporosis, diabetes, patient debilitation, and polypharmacy. The presence of these conditions has been known to compromise the success of osseointegration.

The reasons for tooth loss and presence of uncontrolled periodontal disease and infections have also been implicated in the success or failure of implant. Peri-implantitis, which causes inflammation of supportive tissues around the implants, has been linked to the same bacteria prevalent in periodontal disease.

There are also more internal factors specific to the site of placement, including bone height, bone density, and the amount of attached mucosa. Minimum bone height indicates the need of shorter implants, which has relatively poorer prognosis.

Movable tissue around an implant has also been implicated in inducing the onset of peri-implantitis, which lower the prognosis. The choice of implant type or material plays a role in clinical success. Implant failure has also been associated with immediate loading of the implants as well as implant staging (two-stage versus one-stage).

Other critical factors include implant proximity to the natural teeth and other existing implants.

SUMMARY

Dental implant is the predictable modality for the replacement of lost tooth. However, its prognosis is dependent on the clinician as well as the patient; thus, successful osseointegration is dependent upon proper treatment planning and surgical protocol. Long-term survival on integrated implants needs minimum marginal bone loss, which affected by oral health, hygiene maintenance and external loads on the implants. These loads may be pathological or physiological. Thus, implant's success is multi-factorial and unpredictable. However, proper surgical and prosthodontic protocol in addition to patient compliance may result in long lasting implants.

CHAPTER
14

Occlusal Consideration for Implant Supported Prosthesis

After successful surgical and prosthetic rehabilitation of patient, stresses and loads applied to the implant and surrounding tissues will become a determining factor for success or failure. Complications (prosthetic and/or bony support) may arise because of underlying occlusion. Final factor is the development of an occlusal scheme that minimizes risk factors and allows the restoration to function in harmony with rest of the stomatognathic system.

NATURAL TOOTH VS IMPLANT MOBILITY

The presence of a periodontal membrane around natural teeth significantly reduces the amount of stress transmitted to the bone, especially at the crestal region, and acts as a viscoelastic "shock absorber". It also extend the time in which the load is dissipated. Compared with tooth the direct bone interface with an implant is not as resilient, so that energy imparted by an occlusal force is not partially dissipated. But rather transmits a higher intensity to the contiguous bone.

The mobility of a natural tooth can increase with occlusal trauma. After the occlusal trauma is eliminated, the tooth can return to its original condition with respect to the magnitude of movement. Mobility of an implant can also develop under occlusal trauma. However, after the offending element is eliminated, an implant rarely returns to its original rigid condition. Instead its health is compromised, and failure is usually eminent.

The width of almost every natural tooth is greater than the width of the implant used to replace the tooth so that lesser magnitude of stress transmitted to the surrounding bone. Implant is less effective in resisting lateral (bucco-lingual) bending loads which can concentrate in the crestal region in the jaw. Under similar mechanical loading conditions, implants generate greater stresses and strains at the crest of bone compared with a tooth.

The tooth can show clinical signs of increased stress such as enamel wear facets, stress lines, pits on the cusps of teeth, etc. An implant crown rarely shows clinical signs other than fatigue fracture resulting in significant increases in stress and higher incidence of failure for the other implants in the associated prosthesis.

Teeth benefit from increased occlusal awareness, e.g. premature contact, compare with implants. Implants and teeth also have different proprioceptive information. When implants are subjected to repeated occlusal loads, microscopic stress fractures, work hardening, and fatigue may result.

The natural tooth, with its modulus of elasticity similar to the bone, periodontal ligament, and unique cross sections and dimensions constitutes a near perfect optimization system to handle the stress. An implant handles stress very poorly.

Occlusion on Natural Teeth and Implants

In the implant-tooth fixed prosthesis, four important components may contribute movements to the system: implant, bone, tooth, and prosthesis. The existing occlusion is evaluated and occlusal prematurities are ideally eliminated before implant reconstruction. Unlike teeth, implants do not extrude, rotate, or migrate under occlusal forces.

As such, the restoring dentist may vary the intensity of the force, applied to an implant without causing the implant to readily change its position in bone. On the contrary, natural teeth do exhibit mesial drift, and slight changes in occlusal position do occur over time. The proposed occlusal adjustment does not encourage additional tooth movement because regular occlusal contacts occur. The teeth opposing implants are not taken out of occlusion. Brief occlusal contacts on a daily basis maintain the tooth in its original position.

Implant Orientation and Influence of Load Direction

Implants are designed for a long axis load to the implant body. Stress contours were primarily concentrated at the transosteal (crestal) region. An axial load over the long axis of an implant body generates a greater proportion of compressive stress than tension or shear forces. The greater the angle of load to the implant long axis, the greater the compressive, tensile, and shear stresses. The amount of stress increased with angled load and also type of stress converts to more dangerous shear component, which is conducive to bone loss and has shown to impair successful bone regrowth.

Bone Mechanics and Occlusion

Cortical bone of human long bones has been reported as strongest in compression, 30 percent weaker in tension, and 65 percent weaker in shear. The reported strength of cortical bone decreases with an increasing angle of applied load. The primary component of the occlusal force should therefore be directed along the long axis of the implant body not on angle or following an angled abutment post. Angled abutments are only used only to improve the path of insertion of the prosthesis or the final esthetic result.

Angled load increases the amount of crestal stresses around the implant body, transforms a greater percentage of the force to tensile and shear force, and reduces bone strength in compression and tension. In contrast the surrounding implant body stress magnitude is least and strength of bone is greatest under a load axial to the implant body. All three of these factors mandate the elimination of lateral forces.

Occlusion evaluation and adjustment in partially edentulous implant patients are more important than in natural dentition because the premature contacts can result in more damaging consequences on implants compared with teeth.

Implant Protective Occlusion

Occlusal Table Width

A wide occlusal table favors offset contacts during mastication or parafunction. Wider root form implants can accept a broader range of vertical occlusal contacts while still transmitting lesser forces at the permucosal site under offset loads. Therefore in Implant protected occlusion the width of the occlusal table is directly related to the width of the implant body.

During the mastication, the amount of force used to penetrate the food bolus is also related to the occlusal table width. The wider occlusal table, the greater the force developed by the biologic system to penetrate the bolus of food. Posterior narrow occlusal table combined with reduced buccal contour (in posterior mandible) permits easier sulcular oral hygiene (facilitate daily home care) in a manner similar to a tooth and improves axial loading as well as reduces the risk of porcelain fracture. As a result in nonesthetic regions of the mouth, the occlusal table should be reduced in width compared with natural teeth.

Crown Contour

Whenever possible the portions of an implant crown that are not supported by an axially positioned implant should be recontoured so they do not receive occlusal loads. Alternatively several additional implants should be used to dissipate the force (Figs 14.1 to 14.5).

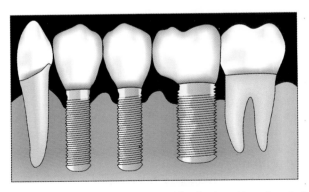

Fig. 14.1: If implant for a molar restoration is placed too close to the adjacent tooth, compromised contours and occlusal table may results

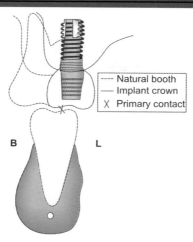

Fig. 14.2: When esthetics are not a concern the distal one-half of the first molar and/or the entire second molar is often resorted in crossbite to improve the direction of forces

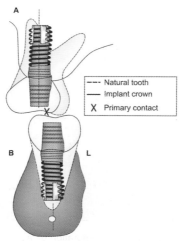

Fig. 14.3: Contours of opposing crown are reduced in width to minimize the occlusal table width and axially load the implants

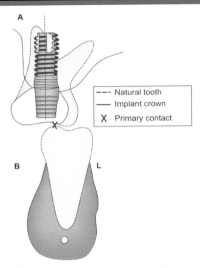

Fig. 14.4: Maxillary implant opposing mandibular natural teeth, the mandibular buccal cusp acts as the primary tooth contact

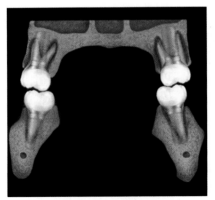

Fig. 14.5: The implants should be placed so that the projection of the fixture is contained within the anticipated crown form

Influence of Surface Area

The adequate surface area should be to sustain the load transmitted to the prosthesis.

Occlusal Materials

Materials selected for the occlusal surface of the prosthesis affect the transmission of forces and the maintenance of occlusal contacts. Occlusal materials may be evaluated by esthetics, impact force, a static load, chewing efficiency, fracture, wear, interarch space requirements and accuracy of castings (Table 14.1).

Table 14.1: Characteristics of three most common groups of occlusal materials are porcelain, acrylic, and metal

	Porcelain	*Gold*	*Resin*
Esthetics	√	×	√
Impact force	×	√	√
Static load	√ ×	√ ×	√ ×
Chewing efficiency	√	√	×
Interarch space	×	√	×
Wear	√	√	×
Fracture	×	√	×
Accuracy	×	√	×

SUMMARY

Occlusion Features in Designing a Fixed Implant-Supported Prosthesis

- Loads should be spread widely, avoiding local high concentration
- We should avoids canine guidance

- With heavy loads optimize the number and position of implants and provide biteguard for night wear.

Occlusion Feature in an Implant Supported Complete Overdenture

- In complete denture there should be balanced occlusion
- Against natural arch we should avoid canine guidance.

Occlusion Feature in the Partially Dentate Patient

The design of occlusion in the partial dentate case requires careful consideration. As we know that the physiologic mobility of natural teeth is absent in the implant, we should avoid transfer of excessive forces to the implants by adjustment of occlusion.

To minimize lateral loads on posterior implant prosthesis, disclusion should occur in lateral and protrusive movements. This may not be possible when a natural canine is to be replaced with prosthesis; however it is recommended that there should be shallow disclusion, and group function should be avoided.

Posterior implant-stabilized prosthesis where a canine is not to be replaced, the occlusion should be arranged to provide:

- Contact of opposing natural teeth
- Multiple light contacts in intercuspal position
- No working or non working interferences.

When canine is to be presents, the occlusion should be arranged to provide:

- Multiple light contacts in intercuspal position
- Opposing natural teeth
- Shallow canine disclusion
- No working or non working interferences.

For anterior bridgework-in these situations the occlusion should be arranged where possible to provide:
- Multiple light contacts in intercuspal position,
- Shallow anterior disclusion shared by the prosthetic teeth.

Occlusion Feature in Single Tooth Implants

In replacing an anterior tooth there should be light occlusal contacts in the intercuspal position, while in protrusive movements these should be smooth, and similar to those on remaining anterior teeth.

If the intercuspal position is not precise or there are multiple missing teeth, then the use of an occlusal rim or jaw registration with acrylic bonnets

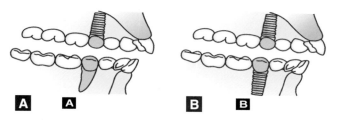

Figs 14.6A and B: (A) When designing on implant crown opposing a natural dentition, light contact in the intercuspal position is preferred while maintaining heavy contact between the adjacent natural dentition. (B) If implant crowns oppose implant crowns, it is preferred that there is little or no contact of these crowns when the patient is in the intercuspal position

will help facilitate the mounting the casts. It is recommended that wherever possible a mutually protected occlusion should be provided. That is scheme in which there are stable occlusal contacts in the posterior part of mouth in intercuspal position (ICP), and where possible no working or nonworking contacts on the implant retained prosthesis. Canine guidance, if present on the natural teeth, should be provided on the implant-stabilized prosthesis (Figs 14.6A and B).

CHAPTER 15

Orthodontic Microimplant

Anchorage management has been a great challenge for orthodontists in every orthodontic treatment. Clinicians continue to need anchorage that displays a high resistance to displacement. Earlier, orthodontists used extraoral traction to reinforce intraoral anchorage. To prevent unwanted tooth displacements in the event of inadequate anchorage potential, orthodontic implants as well as implants serving as prosthetic abutments are used. Prosthetic or endosseous implants have been used successfully for orthodontic anchorage, their clinical applications are still limited in edentulous or retromolar areas because of their size and complicated fixture designs. Other disadvantages include a long waiting period (2-6 months) for bone healing and osseointegration, comprehensive clinical and laboratory work, difficult removal after treatment and high cost. Orthodontic titanium microimplants with specially designed heads that have helped to solve the problems of anchorage control.

INTRODUCTION

The growing demand for orthodontic treatment methods that require minimal compliance and provide maximal anchorage control, particularly by adults has lead to the expansion of implant technology in orthodontics. The ideal intraoral anchorage would not displace, and would require a source devoid of periodontal membrane, which tends to respond to tension and pressure allowing movement through bone. Recently prosthetic osseointregrated implants have been used as

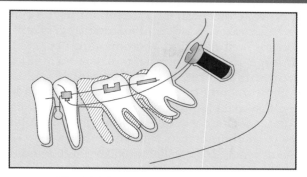

Fig. 15.1: Implant used as a anchorage

intraoral orthodontic anchorage (Fig. 15.1), but their bulky size, complicated fixture designs, long waiting period (4-6 months) for bone healing and osseointegration, comprehensive and clinical as well as laboratory work, difficult removal after treatment, cost and invasiveness have limited their orthodontic application.

The development of small diameters titanium microimplants with specially designed heads that accepts ligatures, coil springs and elastics have helped to solve main objection to previous implants. The titanium microimplant has been designed specifically for orthodontic use and has a button and bracket like head with a small hole that accepts ligatures and elastics. Smaller diameter of 1.2 to 1.8 mm allows its insertion in to many areas of the maxilla and mandible.

Types of Microimplants

Microimplant anchorage are thin, so could be placed intraradicular between the roots, immediate loading with durable mechanical attachment in the cortical bone without the need of osseointegration and important cost friendly. Microimplants are a stable anchorage for orthodontic tooth movement. The microimplant remained stationary under orthodontic loading. Although the screw head was tipped forward significantly 0.4 mm on an average, the displacement would be clinically insignificant. Types of microimplant as follow:

1. *Small head (SH) type:* For maxillary and mandibular attached gingiva including palate.
2. *No head (NH) type:* Maxillary and mandibular soft tissue.
3. *Long head (LH) type:* Mandibular attached gingiva and mucosa border area.
4. *Circle head (CH) type:* Mandibular and maxillary attached gingiva including palate.
5. *Fixation head (FH) type:* Maxillary and mandibular buccal area for intermaxillary fixations.

Types of Surgical Procedures

1. *Open method:* When the head of microimplant is exposed in oral cavity (Fig. 15.2).
2. *Closed method:* When the head of microimplant is embedded under soft tissue, the soft tissue will grow up and embed the microimplant head during treatment. So, in this situation it is better to embed the microimplant under the soft tissue from very beginning of treatment (Fig. 15.3).
3. *Diagonal insertion:* The microimplant is inserted in to the bone in an oblique direction to the bony surface. Microimplant sites need to have a 30-60° angulation to the long axis of teeth both buccally and lingually (Fig. 15.4).

4. *Perpendicular insertion:* Here the microimplant is inserted in the bone in almost perpendicular direction to the bony surface (Fig. 15.5).

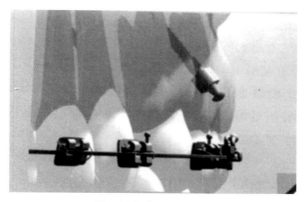

Fig. 15.2: Open method

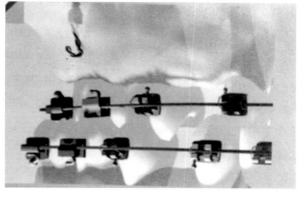

Fig. 15.3: Closed method

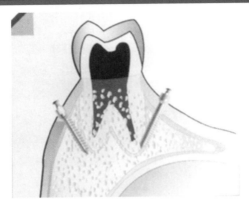

Fig. 15.4: Diagonal insertion

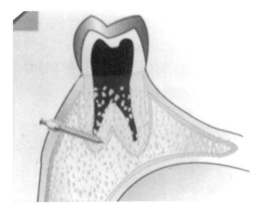

Fig. 15.5: Perpendicular insertion

Selection of Microimplant

1. *Length of microimplant:* A general rule of thumb should be, to use longest possible microimplant, without jeopardizing the health of adjacent

tissues. Recommended size is more than 6 mm in maxilla and 5 mm in mandible.

2. *Diameter of microimplant:* Microimplant with diameter 1.2 mm and 1.3 mm can be used to withstand forces up to 300 g. Microimplant with diameter 1.4 mm, 1.5 mm and 1.6 mm are used when force amount is greater than 300 g. The microimplants with diameter 1.7 mm and 1.8 mm are designed specially for intermaxillary fixation after orthognathic surgery.

Implant Driving Methods

1. *Self-tapping method:* In this method the microimplant is driven into the tunnel of bone formed by drilling, making it tap during implants driving (Fig. 15.6).

2. *Self-drilling method:* In this method the microimplant is driven directly into bone without drilling. This method is used in case of larger diameter implant (Fig. 15.7).

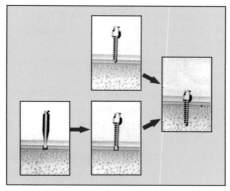

Fig. 15.6: Self-tapping method

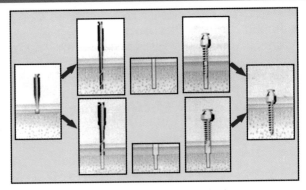

Fig. 15.7: Self-drilling method

Installation Procedures

In most of the buccal/labial applications preference is given to tapered screws -1.3 mm at the head and 1.2 at the tip of varying length depending upon the quality of cortical bone at the site 6-8 mm. They do fat in perfectly between the roots, ideally about a millimeter away from the adjacent roots. Usually achieved by slanting the insertion path of the screws (as the roots taper apically) 30-40 degrees in maxilla and 20-30 degrees in the mandible to the long axis of the teeth. But when it is inserted more apically (in cases where we need intrusion in addition to retraction) in maxillary buccal segments it requires a small vertical stab incision as we encounter free gingival and insertion path has to be more horizontal to avoid the maxillary sinus.

Small amount of local anesthesia is required just to get the numbness of soft tissues only. While anesthetizing palatal mucosa, needle can probe and measure mucosal thickness and help determining microimplant length necessary for anchorage.

A speed reduction contra-angle hand piece is used to make original entry into bone. Make a vertical incision in movable soft tissue, then make a small indentation on bony surface, after this a pilot drill that should be 0.2/0.3 mm smaller than microimplant. A slow drill speed (400-500 rpm) with water irrigation reduces the heat and keeps the surgical site lubricated. Do not use excessive force with the drill. For implant driving both hand and engine drivers are available. Recently to prevent breakage of microimplants during driving a hand driver with built-in torque restrain has been developed.

Force Application

Theoretically we have to wait 2-3 months for osseo-integration between titanium surface and bones. But actually there was no clinical difference in failure rates between immediate loading and delayed loading, if we keep the applied force to less than 300 g.

Palatal Implant

Orthodontic implants have a diameter of 3.3 mm and a length of 4.0 or 6.0 mm is used as palatal implants. Best insertion region in children and adolescent is 4.0 mm distal from the incisive papilla and 3 mm lateral from the palatal midline. Known rare complications include perforation of the nasal cavity and loss through bone resorption, which could be reduced or avoided by correct positioning and sophisticated surgical techniques. The loss rate is less than 15% within the first 3 months. 3-4 month period for integration is recommended. After a period of 6 months for retention, the implant can be removed with stencil drill (Figs 15.8A to C).

Advantage

- Easy to place and remove,
- Orthodontic implants permit maximum anchorage, as well as tooth movements that

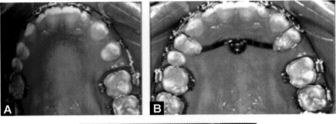

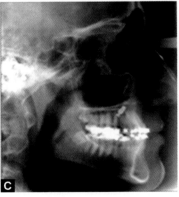

Figs 15.8A to C: (A) Premolar mesialization with pressure springs. (B) Anchorage of the premolars is enhanced by the implant through the transpalatal arch. (C) Lateral cephalogram obtained immediately after insertion of the implant

were previously feasible only with extraoral appliances
- Other advantage of this type of appliance is that it is minimal invasive and
- Duration of treatment of time is shortened.

Disadvantage
- A complex presurgical diagnosis is necessary in some case even before implantation
- Cost of treatment becomes higher
- Some implants should not be inserted under age of 14 years (Especially palatal implant).

The type of implant and anchorage appliance to be used has to be decided after weighting the pros and cons for each individual case. Since osseointegrated implants cannot be loaded until a good interface has formed between implant surface and a bone, a healing period and break in the treatment are involved.

Implant Removal

As with all implant insertions, there is risk of failure, which in case of orthodontic implants, can result from loosening or premature loss of the implant during healing phase or while being used for anchorage purposes. Fortunately strong osseo-integration does not occur between microimplant and bone; this simplifies the removal of these *in-vivo* screws.

Reasons of Failure

Failure of implants is very much a part of this modality- the most common causes are two:

- Root proximity (the jiggling of roots during mastication unseats implant)
- Poor quality of cortical bone at the site, leading to loosening in a few days after insertion. In these instances it is good not to withdraw the implant completely (if that happens it requires anesthesia for new entry). It is good to withdraw partially by few turns, and the reinsert changing the insertion line away from the offending root.

Limitations

- Clinician's skill
- Patient's physical condition
- Site selection
- Patient oral hygiene.

Indications in Orthodontics

Placing microscrew (microimplants) in patients mostly for anchorage conservation whilst retraction and combined with intrusion of anterior teeth when needed. Occasionally it has been used for exclusive intrusion of anterior or posterior teeth, as well as correction buccal crossbites without disturbing the occlusal cant (compared to crossbite elastics). They do remarkable job of distal driving buccal segments-especially when the third molars are missing or extracted. These microimplants anchors seem to have done wonders in terms of sheer amount retraction, in those severe bialveolar/bidental protrusion cases leading to exceptional facial skeletal corrections. More so there is a favorable anticlockwise rotation of mandible even in non growing adults enhancing facial improvements.

SUMMARY

Orthodontic microimplant or miniscrews are cost effective, waiting period for osseointegration not required and they are a stable anchorage for orthodontic tooth movement but do not remain absolutely stationary like an endosseous or prosthetic implant throughout orthodontic loading. Therefore, miniscrews should not be placed at a site adjacent to any vital organ. A suitable implant site for miniscrews could be non-tooth bearing area that has no foramen or pathway for any major nerves and blood vessels. When miniscrews are placed in a tooth bearing area, clearance of 3 mm between the miniscrew and the dental root is recommended. If a prosthetic appliance is to be inserted on completion of orthodontic therapy, interdisciplinary co-operation must start during planning phase.

CHAPTER
16

Complications of Dental Implants

Complications may occur in both the surgical and prosthodontic phase of implants treatments. Most of failures may occur soon after surgical placement or before loading. Failure of osseointegration is relatively rare in well planned cases. It is essential to warn patient of the possibility of surgical and postoperative problems. In most cases complications may be avoidable by careful attention to diagnosis and treatment planning and good surgical and prosthodontic planning.

SURGICAL COMPLICATIONS

It is possible to complications related to surgery may occur e.g. swelling, bruising and discomfort. All patients should be warn of these complications and anticipated extent of them before surgery is undertaken.

As with all minor surgical procedures can be minimized by preoperative, operative and postoperative procedures. Adequate anesthesia, gentle surgical manipulation of both hard and soft tissues, pre and postoperative analgesia, and careful postoperative wound management, including the use of pressure and ice packs to reduce swelling should be properly monitored.

Hemorrhage may occur at the time of surgery if there is excessive trauma to soft tissue or damage to aberrant vessels within the bony cortex. Failure to establish good primary stability at the time of implant placement may result in early failure.

Incorrect positioning of implants at the time of surgery, as a consequence of a poor planning or lack of necessary skills, knowledge and understanding may result in considerable difficulty during the restorative phase of treatment. It is essential to use surgical guides and templates for proper positioning of implants. Use of an appropriate sequence of drills will provide for optimum bone-implant contact, neither too tight nor too loose, and therefore optimize implant location and the achievement of good primary fixation.

Unanticipated Bone Cavities and Indentations

Despite careful radiographic assessment, it may found at surgery that the bone contours are not as anticipated. It may then be necessary to reorient the direction of the implant, and hence that of drills, bearing in mind the type of final restoration. If it is retrievable system, or a screw retained prosthesis, then access hole need to be located in the cingulum or occlusal surface of the prosthetic tooth. Careful knowledge of the selection of abutments available, e.g. angled abutments is important for the surgeon, so that an unanticipated change in implant orientation does not compromise the restorative outcome.

Buccal concavities in the bone can result in some implant threads being exposed. In poor quality of bone the operator may find that the long axis of the site of preparation may veer latterly and it is therefore necessary to use a secure finger rest to avoid this happening. Sometimes we can face problems during seating the implant due to dense bone and is managed by removing the implant and widening the hole with larger diameter drill. Excessive heat can be generated by attempting to fully seat an implant that is proving resistant to placement, and it has been suggested that compression necrosis of the bone may occur as a result.

Failure to achieve primary stability at the time of placement results in a high probability of failure, since initial stability is a virtual prerequisite for osseointegration. The situation may be retrieved by removing the implant and placing one of the slightly larger diameters.

Postoperative Pain

Mild postoperative pain is to be expected. If there are severe pain following surgery (although very rare), patient should be monitored for signs of infection, bleeding and other complications. In such situations there may well be an increased risk of implant failure. The routine use of antibiotics pre and postoperatively will decrease the possibility of infection.

Wound Dehiscence

In the two stage surgical technique, breakdown of the soft tissue following implant placement may lead to the exposure of the implant and cover screw (Fig. 16.1). This may be the result of poor soft tissue coverage of the implant or trauma from prosthesis covering the surgical site. With careful flap design and considerate tissue handling this is rare complication. In all cases the surgical sites must be kept clean with antiseptic mouthwash used as indicated clinically.

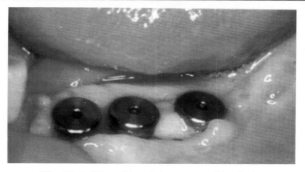

Fig. 16.1: Wound breakdown around implants

Paresthesia

Paresthesia may arise following trauma to nerves in the region of the implant site. The trauma may be direct from drilling through, or at least into a structure or indirect as a result of excess heat generation. Trauma to the sensory nerves may lead to the loss of sensation to the lower lip. Transient loss of sensation in the lower lip may occur from bruising and swelling of soft tissue around the mental foramina. If paresthesia is still present after 2 days, appropriate radiographs may be taken to check for evidence of potential damage to the mandibular or mental nerves. If radiograph do not suggest such a possibility, paresthesia may be associated with the injection of a local anesthetic. This is usually transient, but may last for up to 6-9 months. Damage to the mandibular nerve due to osteotomy preparation or implant placement may be permanent, and specialist advice should be sought.

Mandibular Fractures

In severely resorbed mandibles multiple implants may weaken the jaw with resultant fracture. This is, however, very rare in suitably planned cases.

Complications Following Second Stage Surgery

Second stage surgery involves uncovering of implant, removal of the cover screw, replacing it with a healing abutment and careful suturing of the soft tissues around the abutment. Following complications may occur

- Failure to integrate: Mobility of an exposed implant is indicative of failure of the implant to integrate. The implant and any associated soft tissue should be removed. Either we place larger diameter implant or to leave the site to heal with time to replan treatment
- Excessive bone over the cover screw: Occasionally the cover screw can be partially covered by bone. This bone needs to be cleared away before attempting to remove the cover screw. Most implant systems supply a bone mill for this procedure
- Bone growth between the cover screw and implant: If cover screw has not been placed directly on the implant head at the time of first-stage surgery, Bone may grow into any gap left between implant head and cover screws. Implant systems include a bone mill for the careful removal of bone from the implant head and thereby provide a clear path of insertion for the abutment.

PROSTHETIC COMPLICATIONS

Implant prosthodontics can be relatively uncomplicated when angulation and positioning is ideal. In most cases it can be avoided by means of careful preoperative treatment planning and meticulous attention to detail both clinically and Laboratory.

Biomechanical problems may include:

Fracture of prosthesis (Fig. 16.2A and B)

Fracture of a fixed implant superstructure is often the result of:

- Improper space
- Thin section of material
- Errors in technical procedures
- Generation of excessive stresses in poorly placed prosthesis
- Bond and fatigue failure.

Tooth fracture may be promoted by deterioration in the occlusion. Partial loss of acrylic or porcelain and fracture of the metal framework is more often than the result of excessive loading or poor design of the framework. Long cantilevers can lead to both fracture of the prosthesis and screw loosening. As the fracture of any restoration, cause of the failure

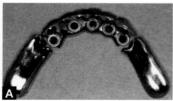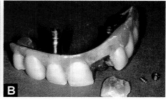

Figs 16.2A and B: (A) Fractured fixed prosthesis (B) Possible causes include mechanical overload, design and fabrication error

must be diagnosed before planning remedial treatment.

Loosening or Fracturing Screws

Overload, poor fit of framework or component and excess or inadequate tightening and poor primary stability in poor quality bone are all reasons for the loosening or fracturing of the screws. Proper protocols must be followed to retrieve and replace fractured screws successfully.

Lute Failure in a Cement-retained Prosthesis

This may happen because of excessive loading and poor fit of the superstructure are the most common cause for this type of failure. Remedial treatment may include repositioning the superstructure to improve fit. Repeated cement failure may necessitate a remark of the prosthesis.

Fracture or Loss of Implants

Bone loss may continue to a level at which inherent weakness in the implant result in fracture. Excessive loading may result in loss of integration. Further treatment under such circumstances is highly dependent on the particulars of the case. Removal of a fracture implant may be problematical.

Physiological problems

- *Appearance:* Problems often reflect bone resorption and resultant disparity in the relationship of the implant to the prosthesis. Soft tissue contours can be difficult to reconstruct, for example as a result of local resorption of alveolar bone. In removable prosthesis problems can arise where implants are inappropriately located

- *Soft tissue inflammation:* Peri-implant mucositis and peri-implantitis
- *Bone loss resulting in implant thread exposure:* Depending on severity of bone loss which may necessitate implant replacement
- *Loss of integration:* Implant removal and perhaps replacement.

A regular programme of monitoring patient complaints of new implant-supported prosthesis is required in order to avoid unexpected difficulties arising from mechanical failure or patient neglect. Patients may complain of new implant prosthesis in a following way.

- Looseness/instability of removable prosthesis,
  - Ensure correct fit and retention of anchorage
  - Assess base extension,
  - Confirm correct jaw relation and occlusion.
- Difficulty with oral hygiene,
  - Disclose and demonstrate plaque accumu-lation.
  - Observe cleaning/brushing techniques of the patient.
  - Arrange repeated hygiene instruction.
- Food accumulation
  - Encourage patient to rinse after meal,
  - Use water jet.
- Speech impairment
  - Speech problems may be associated with changed contours and dead space below fixed prosthesis required for oral hygiene.

- Persistent complain may be solved with flexible obturator inferior to fixed prosthesis, or adjustment of prosthetic space for overdenture.
- Mastication problems
  - Masticatory problems are unusual but can arise with occlusal wear when using implant stabilized fixed prostheses.

CONCLUSIONS

Surgical and prosthodontic complications should be carefully assessed diagnosed and rectified; patient should be informed accordingly for any possible complications prior to treatment. The cause of prosthodontic complications should be carefully monitored.

CHAPTER 17

Maintenance of Dental Implants

A prerequisite to a successful endosteal dental implant should be obtaining a premucosal seal of the soft tissue to the implant surface, as the junctional epithelium provides a seal at the base of sulcus against the penetration of chemical and bacterial substances in natural dentition.

THE PROSTHESIS

Clinical examination of the prosthesis should in addition to checking fit, stability, occlusal relationship and patient acceptability-focus on the status of the patient oral hygiene. Failure or inability of patients to maintain and look after their implant retained prosthesis may lead to many varied problems (Fig. 17.1), including failure in clinical service. The prosthesis and implant abutments should be cleaned by numerous aids. These range from conventional to electric toothbrushes, floss and

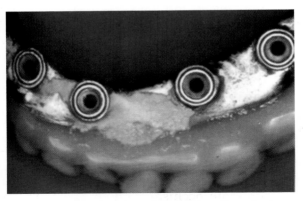

Fig. 17.1: Poor and hygiene. Calculus deposits on the inner surface of prosthesis

superfloss and various interdental brushes and related devices. The patient should be encouraged to maintained a high level of oral hygiene around prosthesis and receive detailed oral hygiene instructions.

Evaluation and maintenance of soft tissue surrounding implant abutments should be both systemic and detailed. Gentle probing should not result in bleeding or exudates. A standard periodontal probe may be used to evaluate probing depths. Most inflammatory conditions can be managed by careful attention to the oral hygiene, aided and supported by professional advice and assistance.

Soft tissue inflammation (mucositis) is sometimes seen around poorly maintained and loose prostheses. Inflamed tissue can be painful, exacerbate the difficulties of oral hygiene, produce an unsightly appearance and result in deepened pockets around the implants. If prosthesis is loose it will be necessary to remove it, clean and replace it in mouth.

Soft tissue proliferation is sometimes seen around poorly designed and ill-fitting super-structures. If such proliferation does not respond to local oral hygiene measures it may be necessary to excise the unwanted tissue, possibly as a part of remedial treatment to replace the superstructure with an appropriately designed, well fitting prosthesis.

Peri-implantitis a peri-implant inflammatory condition resulting in progressive bone loss caused by inappropriate occlusal force in the presence of pathologic bacteria in an unfavorable environment.

A periodontitis like process, peri-implantitis can affect dental implants, and because untreated periondontitis may ultimately lead to the loss of natural teeth, peri-implantitis can result in the loss of dental implants. At this time, substantial evidence supports bacterial plaque as the primary etiologic factor in the loss of both teeth and implants. As in periodontitis around natural teeth, clinical findings around failing implant include marked gingival inflammation, deep pocket formation and progressive bone loss. In well executed and maintained cases peri-implantitis is rarely occurred. Management of peri-implantitis involves;

- Careful assessment of the occlusion in the intercuspal position and eccentric movements
- Examination and cleaning of exposed implant surfaces. If there has been tissue proliferation around implant, this may be needed to remove
- Removal, cleaning and servicing of the restorations may be indicated clinically
- Instruction of the patient in effective oral hygiene procedures
- Monitoring and further oral hygiene and prosthesis maintenance instruction as necessary.

If peri-implantitis persists and progresses despite the above measures, the case should be critically reviewed and, if required, the patient referred for specialist care.

Antimicrobial Treatment

To ensure optimum health around the implant, the following must be accomplished:

- Plaque must be inhibited
- Early microbial population on the tooth/implant surface must be negated
- All existing plaque must be eliminated
- The existing plaque must be altered from pathogenic to nonpathogenic microorganism.

The maintenance of dental implant treatment and the management of problems are linked together, however they are separated in this book in different chapter. Maintenance is started by involving routine checks on integrity of osseointegration and avoidance of any condition that threaten it. Clinical methods for confirming osseointegration is based principally upon following;

- *Radiography:* It provides image in two dimensional but is used routinely to assess bone level around implant and indicate crestal bone loss (normally it should not be more than 0.1 mm per year after first year). Radiographs can also indicates lack of bone implant contact, and more extensive bone loss
- *Probing depths:* These indicate the height of the crestal bone-implant contact and changes will reflect loss of its extent (probing depth of 3-4 mm is often found)
- *Implant mobility:* Currently it has limited routine clinical value for assessing prognosis; marked mobility is diagnostic failure
- *Soft tissues:* It is important to maintain soft tissue health around implants.

Maintenance of Superstructure

Fixed-Tooth Wear

Causes of wear of occlusal surfaces are multiple and relate to material from which the surface has been made, masticatory frequency and loads, dietary habits and chemical damage. Patients with implant stabilized prosthesis can usually generate significantly higher forces on their teeth than occur with conventional removable devices, and as a result tooth wear can be in some cases be very rapid and troublesome. It should be regularly monitored and is to be refurbished.

Removable Superstructure

Maintenance of these is usually confined to rebasing the denture, and/or replacement of the teeth, and adjusting or replacing retainers.

Screws-loosening

Screws should normally need little maintenance; however it is prudent where feasible to check their tightness. It may be loosen due to poor super-structure fit, interaction between joints, excessive off-axis loads. Where the repeated loosening is caused by poor fit then superstructure may need to be remade or modified by sectioning and resoldering.

Cemented Joints

It normally requires no maintenance. Inflammation in the adjacent soft tissues may reflect poor fit or excess cement. Loosening has similar causes to screwed joints plus cement failure possibly as a result of incorrect technique.

ROLES IN IMPLANT MAINTENANCE

Patient Role

- Proper use of brushes (interdental, hand and motorized brushes)

- Use of mouth washes
- Use of flosses, yarns, tapes dipped in chlorihexidine.

Clinical Role

- Check plaque control effectiveness
- Check for inflammatory changes
- Check patient every 3 to 4 months
- Expose radiograph every 12 to 18 months if no pathology is present and is needed if pathology is present
- If superstructure is retrievable, remove and clean every 18 to 24 months (remove and clean abutment also).

SUMMARY

To avoid failure and proper functioning of implant it is essential to maintain the implant prosthesis properly. Maintenance of implant patients should include regular reviews involving radiographic examinations. Patient should be familiar by treating Implant Dentist for the possible consequences related to non cooperation of implants.

CHAPTER
18

The Future

INTRODUCTION

The future of implant dentistry is very encouraging. With continued development of different technologically advancement related to implants it may be anticipated to have a major impact in different branches of dentistry. Some keys area as follows:

Orthodontics

Resistance of dental implants to movement by the application of orthodontic forces has led to use as anchorage for fixed orthodontic therapy, and special implant designs are used for this.

Implants and orthodontics is related in following ways:

1. In space creation-Orthodontist must be fully aware of the room required to place an implants and can create space for placement of implants.
2. Implants including microimplants may be used as anchorage for fixed orthodontics.

Pedodontics

The role of dental implants in the management of younger patient is limited because implants should not be placed until the cessation of growth. Aspect of pediatric dentistry can do a great deal to facilitate implant treatment in patient reaching adulthood, for example.

- Space maintenance
- Retention of traumatized teeth with poor prognosis through to adulthood.

Prosthodontics

Dental implants mainly developed for replacement of missing teeth. The high rate of success achieved

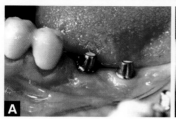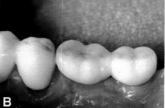

Figs 18.1A and B: (A) Osseointegrated dental implants (B) Fixed prosthesis

with osseointegrated dental implants allowed patient to enjoy the benefits of fixed rather than removable restorations/prosthesis (Figs 18.1A and B).

Periodontics

The relationship between susceptibility to periodontal disease and implants failure remains to be resolved. For placement of implants, it is necessary to maintain proper bone level.

Endodontics

Implants offer a further treatment option to endodontist in managing teeth of poor prognosis. High level of success can be achieved with present day instrumentation and endodontic techniques.

Maxillofacial Surgery

The treatment of maxillofacial defects has been transformed by developments in implantology. Applications for implants in this field continue to expand.

Advances in Implant Dentistry

As concepts of implant dentistry have evolved, there has been an increased emphasis on placing the implant in the correct position relative to the final restoration. Our first advance in refining this process was the use of a surgical template. This device originally was used in conjunction with two-dimensional radiographs. A step forward, but not a perfect answer.

This approach was next fused with computerized tomograms. Specialized software makes it possible to manipulate digitized images of computerized axial tomography (CAT scans) in a computer. It is then possible to plan implant placement digitally. Individual implant can be created, dropped into place, and moved to the appropriate position. Complete digital inventories of most currently available implant systems are stored in the software. This allows those planning the case to see images of the proposed implants and study their relation to each other, the available bone, and contiguous structures.

The advantage of this combined approach is that the case can be preplanned before the case is operated, and in selected situations, the plan can be transmitted to a specialized laboratory that fabricates the surgical template based on the digital plan. There are usually several templates for each case starting with the smallest drill and ending with the largest, thus allowing the operator to be more precise in implant placement.

There are, however, drawbacks, including the time and expense to purchase the software, learning its application, as well as the time needed to plan the case. Technical concerns include making sure that the original tomogram is taken in the correct plane and in a form that is compatible with the software of the planning system. Another serious drawback is found in individuals with metallic restorations, which can create scatter on the tomograms sufficient to make the fabrication of surgical templates using the computer impossible. But the most serious drawback is the operator's inability to "see" the drill inside the osteotomy site.

Thus, even in those cases planned using the software, the surgery is still done blindly. One way of overcoming this problem is the use of real-time imaging technology. This technology, currently in its infancy in dentistry, involves the use of a reference plate that is attached to the patient (usually the arch not receiving surgery) and a second reference plate attached to the implant handpiece. These two reference plates are detected by a "camera" that uses laser technology to relate the position of the patient to the position of the drill. This information is then fed back into a central processing unit that contains a copy of the patient's computerized tomogram. These tomograms are similar to those described above with the exception that a specific reference plate is worn by the patient while the tomogram is taken. This reference plate contains markers that will be used to relate the position of the patient's head and handpiece to the appropriate cut of the patient's CAT scan. It is then possible to see a real-time digital image of the relation of the bur to the patient's osteotomy site during surgery.

RESEARCH

Recent developments in implants have included modifications to surfaces to enhance osseointegration. Efforts will be continue to make the osteo-integration process quicker and even more predictable. Based on sound clinical evidence, more detailed guidelines can be developed that may aid in the improved predictability of dental implants in the special-patient category. Research is ongoing for alternatives to the use of autogenous bone taken from donor sites in the patient. The area includes enhancing bone growth with plasma rich platelets, the use of morphogenic proteins. Further research into other implants materials (e.g. ceramic and ceramic coated implants, polymers, etc.), implants design, implants longevity and cost benefits is set to continue. When the mechanism that ensure implant bioacceptance and structural stabilization are fully understood, implant failure will become a rare occurrence, provided that they are used properly and placed in sites for which they are indicated.

CHAPTER
19

Literature Revisited

Artificial replacement of missing teeth is historical. However, earlier artificial teeth used for substituting the missing natural teeth were extremely poor in appearance and other functions. Humans kept on trying to bring the artificial teeth at par with naturals. Endosseous dental implants are recent attempt for the same. Previous to successful endosseous implants, transmucosal implants and sub-periosteal implants were also attempted.

As per the literature gold was used in the year 1809 in the form of tooth root by Maggiolo. Teeth made of porcelain with lead-coated platinum posts were fitted by Harris in 1887. In the early 1900s' Lambotte fabricated implants of aluminum, silver, brass, red copper, magnesium, gold and soft steel plated with gold and nickel and also characterized corrosion behavior of these metals in body tissues.

The first root form design that differed significantly from the shape of a tooth root was the latticed cage design of Greenfield in 1909, made of iridioplatinum. The surgical cobalt-chromium-molybdenum alloy was introduced in oral implantology in 1938 by Strock.

In 1940, Bothe and his co-workers first reported bone fusing to titanium. Dahl of Sweden proposed the original sub-periosteal implant design and insertion protocol. The first sub-periosteal implant was placed in a patient in US by Gershoff and Goldberg.

Many types of implants were invented by the early-1960s'. Checheve designed a double helical spiral implant made of cobalt-chromium. Clarke and Hickman worked on many metallic biomaterials and found that titanium had maximum passivity. The local tissue response to stainless steel and cobalt-chromium-molybdenum alloys was studied by Mears in 1966. They were found to undergo galvanic corrosion and release metal ions in tissues. Titanium blade implant was introduced in 1968 by Linkow. In the same year a crystalline bone screw was developed by Sandhaus.

In a study on dogs, the use of titanium implants to support the dental prosthesis was first described in 1969 by Branemark et al. Based on his studies, on animals Babbush reported formation of connective tissue around endosseous bladevent implants in 1972. Intramucosal inserts were popularized for the retention of removable maxillary prosthesis in 1974 by Weiss and Judy.

The formation of connective tissue around blade form implants was stated also by Smithloff et al in 1975. Titanium passivates upon contact with air, at room temperature and normal tissue fluids. This is an important property for the consideration of titanium as material for dental implants. Its passivity was reported by Lemons in 1975. Lemons et al studied biocompatibility of surgical grade titanium, cobalt and iron based alloys and selected titanium as the material of choice because of its inert and biocompatible nature paired with excellent resistance to corrosion. Other investigators, including Schroeder in Switzerland, started experiments with titanium endosseous dental implants during the same period of time.

Studies in humans began in 1965 and were followed for 10 years and reported in 1977 by Branemark et al. Sollar and Pollack tested corrosion properties of CP-Ti, Ti-6Al-4V and nitrided Ti-6Al-

4V in Ringer's solution, changing its pH from 1.5 to 9.0, under simulated physiological conditions created by aeration with O_2, N_2 and CO_2, at 37°C, the body temperature. It was inferred from the results that under the most reducing acidic conditions (pH 1.5-1.7, PO_2~0) as might exist in a crevice, Ti-6Al-4V remained passive.

The root form implants were found to be used by ancient Chinese 4000 years ago, Egyptians 2000 years ago, Incas 1500 years ago as per the report of Anjard in 1981. The reactions of bone, connective tissue and epithelium to endosteal implants with titanium sprayed surfaces were studied by Schroeder et al in 1981. The surface modification of titanium was found to have a positive influence on living tissues.

Adell et al published their 15 years clinical case report in 1981 on the use of implants in completely edentulous jaws. 90 percent of the reported anterior mandibular region implants survived 5-12 years later. Lower survival rates were observed in maxilla. They determined that after the first year on average 0.1 mm bone loss was observed in each following year. The use of stainless steel was discontinued because they had galvanic potentials and corrosion tendency (Lucas et al). Cobalt-chromium alloys were discontinued because they exhibited least ductility of all the alloy systems used for dental surgical implants (Lucas et al).

In the anterior mandible non-submerged implant placement and immediate loading of implants was suggested by Ledermann et al in 1982. In a theoretical model, Skalak convincingly demonstrated in 1983 that resinous occlusal surfaces were indicated to prevent traumatic shock-type forces from affecting the health and longevity of the osseointegrated interface. In that model it was postulated that metallic or ceramic occlusal surfaces could transmit substantial impact forces to the osseointegrated interface, putting it at risk for damage and eventual failure. This was the rationale against the use of ceramic occlusal materials for implant supported prostheses.

It was observed by Blomberg and Linquist in 1983 that the osseointegrated implants had a positive effect on the well-being of patients. Yue et al observed in 1984 in a study on porous coated Ti alloy that the porous surface layer was only 70 percent dense in comparison to bulk of the alloy Ti-6Al-4V, and thus its modulus of elasticity was reduced to approximately 30 percent, that of the full density alloy. Lee and Welsch in 1984 recorded variation of young's modulus of Ti-6Al-4V in the range of 108 to 118 GPa, depending on the heat treatment and oxygen concentration.

Roberts et al found in 1983 that strain will not dissipate to the surrounding bone on subsequent orthodontic shifting or relaxation of implants and could negatively affect the survival of dental implants. As reported by Rams et al in the year 1984, the microflora in an implant sulcus is similar that of a natural tooth.

Lundquist et al in a report in 1984 on occlusal perception, stated that implant patient can determine 50 μm differences with rigid implant bridges, compared with 100 μm in those with complete dentures and 20 μm between natural teeth. Lang et al reviewed the possible influences of aluminum and vanadium biodegradation products on local and systemic tissue responses for the perspectives of basic sciences and clinical applications. As per the teachings of Branemark submerged, undisturbed healing was a prerequisite for successful osseointegration. The success of osseointegration in the management of completely edentulous jaws, on long-term effects of chewing on mandibular fixed prostheses is well studied and documented by Lindquist et al in 1985.

The first instance of the dental implant has been recorded in 1565, when the repair of developmental defect of a palate was done using gold, as quoted by Lemons et al in the year 1986. The core vent implant, a hollow basket implant with threaded components to engage bone, was introduced by Niznic in 1986. Babbush gave a protocol in 1986 for the blade form implants which included fabrication of interim implant supported prosthesis on the day of surgery.

Success criteria for endosteal implants were proposed in 1986 by Albrektsson et al. According to him, a successful individual, unattached implant is immobile when tested clinically, a radiograph does not demonstrate any evidence of peri-implant radiolucency and vertical bone loss is less than 0.2 mm annually following the first year of service of implants. Individual implant performance is characterized by absence of persistent and/or irreversible signs and symptoms such as pain, infection, neuropathies, paresthesia, or violation of the mandibular canal. Success rates of 85 percent at the end of 5 years period of observation and

80 percent at the end of 10 years period of observation have been given as minimum criteria for the success.

Steflik did clinical trials in 1986 on single crystal sapphire endosteal implants and clinically observed that rigid fixation needs atleast a portion of implant in direct contact with bone, although the percentage of bone contact cannot be specified. In a study of patient's reactions to jaw bone anchored prosthesis by Albrektsson et al in 1987, 80 percent of the patients judged that their overall psychologic health improved compared with their previous state of wearing traditional, removable prosthodontic devices, and perceived the implant supported prosthesis as an integral part of their body. It was stated by Smithloff et al in 1987 on the basis of their 15 years of study on the use of blade implants that blade implants have low survival rates.

Tatum introduced Omni implant system in 1988. Omni-R is a titanium alloy root form implant with horizontal pins designed to be placed into prepared or expanded endosseous reception site. Another implant introduced by Tatum was Omni-S. The soft tissue interface of dental implants was studied by Meffert in 1988. He found that there was a close adaptation of circular fibers encircling the implant neck. The response of bone to the unloaded and occlusally loaded Core vent and Biotes implants at the light microscopic level, by using non human primate model, was studied by Lum et al in 1988. Histologic examination revealed that both implants achieved osseointegration and maintained the direct contact with bone after 5 months of occlusal loading.

One of the most important innovations in custom implant abutment design was ULCA abutment, created by Lewis et al in 1988. It allows fabrication of custom abutments for use in difficult situations when space is tight or when implant angulation is less than ideal. In the same year, Stefani gave a report on the care and maintenance of the dental implant patient.

Koth et al made a 5 year clinical study on aluminium oxide endosteal dental implant. They found that implants had compatibility with associated bone and soft tissues which correlated with biocompatibility of animal studies. Statistically 77.7 percent of all implants placed, 99.5 percent of these implants were used to support prosthesis. An interesting case report by using custom cast titanium implants to correct alveolar ridge deformities was given by Block et al in 1988. In the year 1989, Schmitt and Zarb gave the criteria for the success of osseointegrated endosteal implants. They suggested patient comfort, sulcus depth, gingival status, damage to adjacent teeth, violation of the maxillary sinus, mandibular canal, or floor of the nasal cavity to consider as criterion.

Van Steenberghe in 1989 evaluated the prognosis of the osseointegration technique applied for the rehabilitation of partially edentulous jaws in a multicenter retrospective study. The observation time varied from 6 to 36 months after prosthetic reconstruction. The success rate for the individual implants in the maxilla and mandible were 87 percent and 92 percent respectively.

In a preliminary study on 876 consecutively placed implants Jemt et al in 1989 reported a successful survival rate in partially edentulous patients. Several authors such as Lundgren et al, Falk et al made empirical recommendations for the length of cantilever extensions of the implant supported full arch fixed prosthesis and the number of teeth that could be cantilevered posterior to the terminal implant. The IMZ concept was introduced by Kirsch and Ackermann in 1989 and was presumed to provide protective, force dampening abutment or "intermobile element" beneath the restoration.

In clinical report of 1989, Zarb and Schmitt stated that 49 dental arches were successfully treated with 44 implants supported fixed partial dentures and 5 implant supported overdentures. The 89.5 percent longitudinal success of individual implants was accompanied by a 100 percent success rate of comfortable and ongoing prosthetic wear.

The role played by forces and strains on the long-term stability and success of the osseointegrated implants has been reported by Rangert et al in 1989. A review by Bruggenkate et al in 1990 stated that the most common clinical criterion reported is the survival rate or whether the implant is still physically in the mouth or has been removed. In a study by Zarb and Schmitt in 1990, 257 implants were placed in 49 dental arches - 43 mandibles and 6 maxillae. After 4-9 years of insertion of implants, 244 or 89.05 percent remained osseointegrated. Of 262 implants in the place more than 5 years, 232 or 88.5 percent were still integrated. Component loosening and fracture have been found to be the common complications of functional loading and overloading of implants (Zarb and Schmitt 1990). From observations of a number of HA coated cylindrical integral implants exhibiting morbidity, Block and Kent in 1990 made recommendations to reduce complications including (i) caution in placing implants in thin bone or extraction sites without adequate bone coverage or grafting and (ii) primary closure to prevent premature exposure and possible bone loss.

Misch stated in 1990 that implant dentistry is expanding. It will continue until every restorative practice uses implants for abutment support of both fixed and removable prosthesis. Ahlquist et al studied osseointegrated implants in 50 edentulous jaws during 2 years of observation period. The implant survival rate was found to be 89 percent in maxilla and 97 percent in mandible. A study by Gammage et al was done on the probing depths between healthy implants with and without coronal collars in 1990. They did not find any significant difference between the implants with and without collars. Studies on osseous healing around the implant were done by Pilliar et al in 1991. They suggested that crestal remodeling is limited to smooth region of the collar.

Kapur in 1991 compared treatment assessment made by two groups of patients. They were fixed partial denture patients supported by bladevent implants and removable partial denture patients. He found that fixed partial denture patients had greater patient satisfaction than the removable partial denture patients.

The periotest is a computerized mechanical device developed by Schulte in 1985. It measures the dampening effect or degree of attenuation against objects by developing a force of 12-18 Newton. The recordings range from –8 to +50, which helps to evaluate the slight changes in rigidity of implant fixation. It was given by Berglundh et al. Teerlinck et al in 1991 found that the bone density around the implant could be correlated with these numbers.

Heimke et al in 1992 discussed the engineering aspects of isoelasticity. They state that, if a close bone contact has to be achieved and maintained, the bond at the bone-implant interface must be strong to withstand all shear forces. Isoelasticity results in similar deformation patterns on loading, preventing shear fracture at implant-host tissue "osseointegrated" interface. Andersson et al in 1992 observed 100 percent survival rate in a prospective study of 37 implants, restored with single crowns. However, once the crowns were loaded, the survival rate was reduced to 94.6 percent after one year. Kononen et al in 1992 reported the effect of surface modification of titanium on the attachment of human gingival fibroblasts (HGF). The cell shape orientation and proliferation of HGF appear to depend on the oxide layer and adjacent bulk material.

The American Dental Association Council on Dental Materials, Instruments and Equipment (1993) has given criteria for the evaluation of implants as (i) durability (ii) bone loss (iii) gingival health (iv) pocket depth (v) effect on adjacent teeth (vi) function (vii) esthetics (viii) presence of infection, discomfort, paresthesia or anesthesia (ix) intrusion on the mandibular canal and (x) patient emotional and psychological attitude and satisfaction.

Removable implant overdenture was found to be suitable for treatment of edentulous maxilla. However fixed or fixed detachable prosthesis was successful in the mandible. It was reported by Boer in 1993. In the same year, Prestipino et al reported the use of high strength ceramic abutments to support crowns. It increased the possibility of esthetic restoration of dental implants. Implant prosthesis components have many complications. In 1993, Kohavi evaluated mechanically and clinically the complications of these implant prostheses components. Loosening of components and their fracture was found on functional loading. In 1993 Wehrbein et al have concluded based on experimental study in dog, that static load does not have adverse effect on osseointegrated implants, when they are used for orthodontic anchorage.

In 1993, Zarb and Schmitt studied prospective results of osseointegrated implants placed in partially edentulous areas in the posterior zones. 105 implants were placed in 46 edentulous areas in 35 patients. After a period of loaded service ranging from 2.6 to 7.4 years (mean 5.2 years), of the 41 implants placed in the maxilla, 40 (97.6%) remained in function, and of the 64 placed in mandible, 59 (92.2%) remained in function. The overall survival rate was 94.3 percent. Also, Zarb and Schmitt reported in 1993 an average success rate of 91.5 percent for implants in anterior part of the partially edentulous mouths both in the maxilla and mandible.

Breme in 1995, in a review on metallic biomaterials, reproduced values for young's modulus, percentage elongation, 0.2 percent offset yield strength, fatigue strength and hardness. He observed that titanium and its alloys possessed the best combination of all these properties. Engquist et al have reported in 1995 after a 1-5 years retrospective study of 82 single tooth endosseous implants, that two implants were best before loading with an overall surgical survival rate of 97 percent. The bone loss averaged 0.9 mm in the first year and then 0.1 mm in each consecutive year. Benson stated in 1995 that the use of dental implants to replace the form and function of the lost natural dentition has become a significant treatment option after dental implant assessment.

Reiser et al stated in 1995, "implant periapical lesion" as implant associated osteolysis occurring after the overheating of bone, implant contamination, or adjacent tooth associated peri-apical infection. In a prospective study Zarb and Schmitt stated that an endosteal implant can maintain bone width and height so long as the implant remains healthy. Preliminary outcomes of the treatment with Branemark single tooth implant supported prostheses, inserted at the University of Toronto, were reported in 1996 by Avivi-Arber et al. A similar study by Henry et al in 1996 indicated promising performance in different jaw locations with a survival rate of 96.6 percent in the maxilla and 100 percent in the mandible. Breeding et al in 1996 evaluated initial retention of Hader clips on an implant bar. They suggested that the greatest changes in initial retention occurred within the first pull separation of the bar-clip retained removable prostheses. Engelman in 1996 stated that the implants should provide improved retention, and support, against displacement. It will reduce the necessity for palatal tissue coverage, while planning for implant supported removable prosthesis.

Tarnow et al and Schintmann et al have reported promising results with implants after immediate loading. Petropoulous et al in 1997 evaluated relationship between the degree of retention and time of release of implant overdenture retention. They compared two implant mandibular overdentures with bar and clip, direct ball attachment, zest attachment, or magnet and keeper. Sauberlich et al in 1998 have done in vitro biocompatibility studies. They have reported that differentially modified titanium surfaces enhance biocompatibility.

The surface microtexture was found to influence the attachment and growth of human gingival fibroblasts (HGF). Surface microstructures were created on titanium surfaces blasting with TiO_2 particles and fibroblasts grown were studied by Mustafa et al in 1998. There was found to be promotion of growth and attachment of HGF.

An overdenture prosthesis supported by two implants was studied by Bergendal and Engquist in 1998. They reported the clinical function and long-term prognosis of overdentures.

Kuboki et al in 1999 compared the quality of life (QOL) level among implant denture, removable partial denture, and no restoration patients with distal extension type unilateral mandibular edentulism. QOL of dental implant patients were higher than those of removable partial denture or no restoration patients. The QOL levels of removable partial dentures patients were almost identical to those of no restoration patients.

Zitzmann et al in their report in 1999 introduced the criteria for planning implant treatment. They included the crucial factors involved in deciding whether a fixed or removable prosthesis should be placed in the edentulous maxilla. In a clinical report Drago in 1990, described the treatment of malocclusion of 49 years old patient, using osseointegrated implants for orthodontic anchorage. Titanium implants were placed in the posterior mandibular edentulous segments. After osseo-integration of implants, standard orthodontic brackets were cemented on to the two-piece temporary healing abutments and were used as anchorage. A study by Koele et al in 1991 assessed, whether dental general practitioners attach to psychosocial patient characteristics during the judgement of suitability of these patients for dental implant treatment. There was a substantial disagreement between what dentists say to be important characteristics and the characteristics they actually used to judge.

Longitudinal peri-implant clinical responses in the mandible were monitored by Richard et al in 1994. They found that peri-implant mucogingival cuffs with relatively deep pocket probing depths inconsequential to the maintenance of bone support around the tested implants. Almog et al in 1999 analyzed the amount of deviation between the planned prosthetic trajectory and residual bone trajectory in different areas of the maxillary and mandibular dental arches. It was done using a tomographic survey in conjunction with imaging/surgical guides. The discrepancies were greater in the mandibular molar area and other sites were not significantly different. Binon in his article in 2000 indicated that more than 90 root form implants are available "in a variety of diameters, lengths, surfaces, platforms, interfaces and body designs".

The analysis of various implant surfaces was done by Orsini et al in 2000. According to them, osteoblast like cells adhering to the machined implants present very flat configuration. The same cells adhering to the sandblasted and acid-etched surfaces show an irregular morphology and pseudopodi. These morphologic irregularities are found to improve initial cell anchorage. This provides better osseointegration for sandblasted and acid-etched implants.

Laser treated titanium surface was studied by Gaggl et al in 2000. The optimal surface structure with least contamination was obtained after laser treatment. A 5 year retrospective study was done by Vigolo et al in 2000 using mini-implants (3i implant innovation, Inc). They reported a survival rate of 94.2 percent. The mini implants for single tooth restorations are found to be suitable in limited spaces where the standard or wide diameter implants are difficult to use. Becker and Kaiser have given in 2000 the indications for the implants to support cantilevered fixed partial dentures. According to them in clinical situations such as implant alignment problems, treatment requiring extensive bone grafting, restricted esthetics, to bypass a deficient site and in location of a failed implant, implant can be cantilevered. A pilot study was made by Gartner et al in 2000, on masticatory muscle coordination between partially edentulous patients restored with implant supported fixed prostheses and control patients. During the maximal occluding force measurement, EMG was done. The masticatory muscle coordination pattern in the implant group showed a tendency to activate the working and non-working side muscles simultaneously. They concluded that patients with implant supported prostheses are well adapted to perform habitual masticatory functions. They also found that on non-habitual function such as maximal occluding force, there was a less coordinated muscle activity.

Certain principles for splinting of implants were given by Becker et al in 2000. They suggested avoiding splinting of implants as far as possible. Splinting of implants to natural tooth was advised when the teeth need support such as a periodontally compromised tooth. They should be provided with an interface attachment in a keyway style, tube locks or A-splints. If splinting is desirable for cross-arch stabilization, not more than 2 to 4 units are advised. Perizzolo et al reported in 2001 that hydroxyapatite and titanium coated micro-machined surfaces accelerate osseous healing. An overall improvement in the bone-implant interface was found producing better osteogenesis. In addition, an interaction between the chemistry and topography was reported. Gross et al examined in 2000 the stress distribution around the implants in a 2-dimensional photoelastic anatomic model. The highest principal stress concentration was seen at the buccal concavity of the maxillary implant. They suggested preservation of the buccal supporting bone volume. It helps to obtain a physiological modeling response to enhance the facial plate.

Cruz et al described in 2001, implant induced bone expansion procedure. It was found to facilitate the placement of implants in atrophic alveolar ridges. Bone expansion was done using wedge-shaped

(Bioform) implants. Kuphasuk et al studied the corrosion behavior of titanium and titanium based alloys at 37°C in Ringer's solution in 2001. They found that all samples showed good corrosion resistance to electrochemical corrosion over the potential of relevance for intraoral conditions. All titanium alloys were covered mainly with rutile type oxide (TiO_2) after corrosion tests. A prospective study was done by Hwan et al in 2001 using Sargon implants, the expandable implant design. Overall survival rate was 96.0 percent in maxilla and 94.8 percent in mandible. Implants placed in fresh extraction sockets showed 98.9 percent survival rate. Healed sites showed 93.9 percent survival rate. Immediate loading of 52 fresh extraction socket implants in the maxilla showed a 100 percent survival rate during the evaluation period of 40 months.

Sadowsky analyzed in 2001, the existing mandibular overdenture literature. It was in relation to bone preservation, effect on antagonist jaw, number of implants required, anchorage systems, maintenance and patient satisfaction. Twelve treatment concepts were elucidated by him in his review. Abron et al studied implant surfaces with ideal pit morphology in 2001. They were found to possess a calculated biomechanical significance. It was found to enhance bone formation in early periods after placement in rat tibia model.

Finite element analysis is commonly used now-a-days. Geng et al has reviewed in 2001, the use of it in relation to the bone-implant interface, the implant prosthesis connection, and multiple implant prostheses. It is found to be used in prediction of biomechanical performance of dental implant systems.

Correction of implant position was given in a clinical report by Poggio et al in 2001. The unesthetic implant position resulted from unexpected post-pubertal growth was corrected by surgical implant repositioning. This was a technique similar to single tooth osteotomies. Chaffee et al illustrated in 2001 difficulties associated with resolving periapical infections of teeth and implants. In vitro study by Williams et al in 2001 evaluated the retentive characteristics of 5 different overdenture designs on 4 maxillary implants. The mean initial retention values ranged from 5.06-19.14 lb. The highest retention value was recorded for the combined ERA/Harder clip design and the lowest for the 2 Harder clip designs. The retention of all designs decreased over the course of 10 consecutive pulls.

In 2002, Proussaefs et al studied the implant which was retrieved after 13 years of service. On examination no obvious signs of HA dissolution was found, called into question the idea that HA-coated implants are susceptible to degradation or dissolution under long-term function. After microscopic analysis of a retrieved implant, Proussaefs in 2002 suggested that HA coating can resist degradation in contact with bone. However, HA was found to be prone to dissolution in contact with soft tissue.

Haas in 2002 used a modified technique to fabricate a long-span fixed prosthesis delivered after serial extractions and implant placement, in a patient with scleroderma. Endosteal dental implants are also used in patients with ectodermal dysplasia. A prospective clinical trial by Gukes et al in 2002 support the continued use of endosteal dental implants in these patients. Appropriate precautions in the maxilla have been advised by them.

Distribution of bone strain on implants was studied by Yacoub et al in 2002. They stated that bone strain resulting from dental implant loading is distributed to adjacent cortices and also to areas distant from dental implants. Larger diameter implants were found to facilitate stress transfer to cortical bone than the small diameter implants. Watanabe et al in 2002 reported effective removal of a malpositioned mandibular implant with a trephine bur followed by a replacement implant.

Celar et al in 2002, in a clinical report have presented the correction of infrapositioned osseointegrated implants in an adolescent female with ectodermal dysplasia and oligodontia with the use of distraction osteogenesis. The distraction was controlled by prosthesis. Rungcharassaeng et al in 2002 studied the peri-implant response of immediately loaded, HA coated implants and conventional, delayed loaded implants after 1-year. Both responses were favorable. According to Sahiwal et al, all the nonthreaded and threaded endosseous implants can be recognized from radiographs made between −100 and +100 vertical inclinations.

Simon in 2002 presented a technique for the fabrication of a surgical and radiographic template, supported by transitional implants. It guides the placement of conventional implants. The template enhances the accuracy of implant placement in an efficient way to achieve predictable esthetic results. A 5-year prospective study by Gibbard and Zarb gave a stable long-term results with single Branemark implant supported crowns. A mean vertical bone reduction of less than 0.2 mm annually was found. In vitro study by Guichet et al in 2002 suggested that excessive contact tightness between the crowns can lead to a non-passive situation. Also splinted restorations exhibit better load sharing to implants than non-splinted restorations.

Gronet et al in 2003 presented a method for the fabrication of acrylic cranial implants for 2 patients. Anatomic modeling technology was used for the fabrication. In 10 years retrospective study by Simon reported in 2003, 49 patients with 126 implants were restored with molar and premolar crowns. The implant failure rate was 4.6 percent. The complications of abutment screw loosening (7%) and loss of cement bond (22%) was recorded. A study was made by Kronstrom et al in 2003 on early functional loading of conical implants in anterior mandible. Implant survival rate of 93 percent with average bone loss of 0.24 mm was recorded by them.

Altard et al reported in 2003, an overall implant survival rate of 91.6 percent and prosthesis survival of 89 percent after 15 years of study on the posterior zones of both the maxilla and mandible. Laster et al introduced a new tricortical implant "Excalibur" in 2003. It is intended for use in posterior maxilla when only 8 mm or less of the resorbed alveolar ridge was present. As per the study of Bryant and Zarb, elders do not have greater bone loss around oral implants in edentulous jaws compared with young adults. Goodacre et al stated in 2003, the most common implant complications like loosening of the overdenture retentive mechanisms (33%), implant loss in irradiated maxilla (25%), hemorrhage - related complications (24%), resin veneer fracture with fixed partial dentures (22%), implant loss with maxillary overdentures (21%), overdentures needing to be relined (19%), implant loss in type IV bone (16%), and overdenture clip/attachment fracture (16%).

Scarano et al in 2003 did in vivo human study using the titanium surfaces coated with titanium nitride (TiN) and found that it reduced bacterial colonization compared to other clinically used implant surfaces. They also found to support fibroblast growth reported by Groessner et al in 2003. Schliephake et al reported in 2003 that HA coated implants exhibit bioreactive surface structure. HA coated implants were found to lead more rapid osseous healing in comparison with metal implants, based on a study on dogs.

Ibanez et al in 2003 studied performance of double acid etched surface external hex titanium implants in relation to one and two stage procedure and found that these implants have relatively high success rates.

Carmine in 2003 studied spreading of epithelial cells on machined and blasted titanium surfaces. A total of 10 machined, 10 sand blasted discs and 10 glass cover slips were used for this study. Samples were analyzed using SEM and the cell spreading area was determined.

It was observed that after 24 hours incubation, keratinocytes grown on sand blasted titanium samples displayed numerous long and branched or dendritic filopodia closely adapted to surface roughness. While cells cultured on machined surface do not present such cytoplasmic extension and have round morphology. This shows that sand blasted surfaces are the optimal substrate for epithelial cell adhesion and spreading.

Stefano Guizzardi et al in 2004 studied that different titanium surfaces affect osteoblast response. He used six Ti disks with different treatments (i) Smooth surface (ii) Al_2O_3 sand blasted (C150) with acid etching (iii) ZrO_2 sand blasting (B60) with acid etching (iv) ZrO_2 sand blasting (B120) with acid etching.

Surface characteristics were determined by SEM observation and a roughness tester. Raman spectroscopy was used to check residues. Cells were seeded and observed under SEM and growth curve generated with cell counter. Alkaline phosphate activity was also checked.

Results show B60 and B120 surfaces with best surface area contact while smooth surface being poorest. Al_2O_3 debris remains on surface which is toxic to cells.

Abe Y et al in 2005 studied a new biochemical surface modification technique for implants using phosphor-amino acid. Based on the results of this study it was concluded that P-thr (O-Phospho-L-threonine) chemically bonded to the titanium surface treated with HCl.

Phay YM, Tan BT in 2005 did rehabilitation of the edentulous mandible with implant supported over-dentures using prefabricated telescopic coping.

Porter JA, Van Fraunhofer JA in 2005 reviewed the literature concerning the success or failure of dental implants. According to them the main predictors for implant success are quantity and quality of bone, the patient's age, the dentist's experience, location of implant placement, length of implant, axial loading and oral hygiene maintenance. Primary predictors for failure are poor bone quality, chronic periodontitis, systemic diseases, smoking, unresolved caries or infection, advanced age, implant location, short implants, accentric loading and inadequate number of implant, para functional habits and absence/loss of implant integration with hard tissues. Inappropriate prosthesis design also may contribute to implant failure.

Levin L, Schwartz Arad D in 2005 studied the effect of cigarette smoking on dental implants and related surgery. Cigarette smoking may adversely affect wound healing and thus jeopardize the success of bone grafting and dental implantation. Heat as well as toxic byproducts of cigarette smoking such as nicotine, corbon monoxide, hydrogen cyanide have been implicated as risk factors for impaired healing and may effect the success of surgical procedures.

Thor A, Wannfors K in 2005 did a controlled clinical study to evaluate whether PRP (Plasma Rich-Plasma) in conjunction with grafting of particulated autogeneous bone to the maxilla could improve the integration and clinical function of dental implants. Nineteen consecutive patients were included in the study and treated with iliac bone grafts and dental implants in maxilla according to a split mouth design. In anterior maxilla, particulated bone mixed with PRP (test) was compared with onlay block grafts without PRP (control). In posterior maxilla, particulated bone grafts with (test) or without (control) PRP were placed as sinus inlay grafts. After 6 months of healing; 152 implants were placed. Test (PRP; 76 implants) and non-PRP (76 implants) sites were evaluated and compared by implant survival rate, marginal bone level, and implant stability using resonance frequency analysis RFA during one year in function. The present clinical study showed that a high implant survival rate and stable marginal bone conditions can be achieved after 1-year of loading in the maxilla following autogeneous bone grafting whether or not PRP is used, only with use of PRP, handling of particulated bone grafts was improved.

Fischer K, Stenberg T in 2006 carried out a randomized controlled trial to compare biologic and technical treatment outcomes and patient satisfaction after early loaded implants with those of implants loaded after a healing period of 3 to 4 months in the edentulous maxilla. 24 patients with completely edentulous maxillae were randomized into a test group (n=16) and a control group (n=8). All patients received 5 or 6 solid screw type titanium implants with sandblasted, large grit, acid etched surfaces. Clinical assessments were obtained at loading and other 3,6,12,24,36 months. The cumulative implant success rate 3 years after loading was 100 percent. At the 3-year examination the mean ($P <$ or $= 0.005$), distal ($P <$ or $= 0.005$) and mesial $P > 0.05$) crestal bone levels were better in the test group. No significant differences were noted for any other outcome measure.

Pramono C in 2006 described a partial denture surgical template technique with tube technique using a coen's drill guide, to achieve implant placement parallelism; in combination with a mathematical equation to find the clinical-radiographic discrepancy which can be used as an alternative method in placement guidance of dental implant insertions and its fixed prosthetic treatment planning in a wide edentulous area.

Nirit Tagger Green in 2002 reported fracture of a dental implant, four years after loading. The failure analysis of the implant revealed that the fracture was caused by metal fatigue and that the crown-metal, a Ni-Cr-Mo alloy exhibited corrosion.

Yokoyama et al in 2002 studied the delayed fracture of titanium dental implant. It was concluded that titanium in a biological environment absorbs hydrogen and this may be the reason for delayed fracture of a titanium implant.

Notable changes due to galvanic coupling have been reported in the literature.

Pourbaix in 1984 reviewed the methods of electrochemical thermodynamics (electrode potential-pH equilibrium diagrams) and electro-chemical kinetics (polarization curves) to understand and predict the corrosion behavior of metals and alloys in the presence of body fluids. A short review of the literature is given by Pourbaix concerning some applications of such methods, both *in vitro* and *in vivo*, relating to surgical implants (stainless steels, chromium-cobalt-molybdenum alloys, titanium and titanium alloys) and to dental alloys (silver-tin-copper amalgams, silver-base and gold base casting alloys, nickel-base casting alloys).

The galvanic corrosion of titanium in contact with amalgam and cast prosthodontic alloys has been studied in vitro (Ravnholt, 1988, Geis-Gerstorfer et al 1989; Ravnholt and Jensen, 1991; Strid et al 1991). No current or change in pH was registered when gold, cobalt chromium, stainless steel, carbon composite or silver palladium alloys were in metallic contact with titanium. Changes occurred when amalgam was in contact with titanium.

Geis-Gerstorfer et al in 1994, stated that the galvanic corrosion of implant/superstructure systems is important in two aspects; (i) possibility of biological effects that may result from the dissolution of alloy components and (ii) the current flow that results from galvanic corrosion may lead to bone destruction.

In another study Reclaru and Meyer in 1994 examined the corrosion behavior of different dental alloys, which may potentially be used for superstructures in a galvanic coupling with titanium. Reclaru revealed from his investigations that from electrochemical point of view, an alloy that is potentially usable for superstructures in galvanic coupling with titanium must fulfill the following requisites:

1. In coupling the titanium must have weak anodic polarization.
2. The current generated by the galvanic cell must also be weak.
3. The crevice potential must be much higher than the common potential.

Johanson in 1995 studied the effect of surface treatments and electrode area size on the corrosion of cast and machined titanium in contact with conventional and high copper amalgams in saline solutions with and without fluoride ions. He found that conventional amalgam corroded more than high copper amalgams in contact with titanium in saline solutions and concluded that surface preparations and fluoride affect the electrochemical activity of titanium.

Cortada et al in 1997 had reported that metallic ion release in artificial saliva of titanium oral implants coupled with different metal super-structures. In this work metallic ion release in oral implants with superstructures of different metals and alloys used in clinical dentistry has been determined. This study has been realized in a saliva environment at 37°C. The measurements of the ions released were carried out by means of the Inductively Coupled Plasma Mass Spectrometry technique. The titanium oral implant coupled with a chromium-nickel alloy releases a high quantity of ions and the implant coupled with the titanium superstructure presents a low values of ions release.

From the current literature and experimental study, Venugopalan, and Lucas in 1998 defined the profile for an acceptable couple combination as:
1. The difference in OCP (open circuit potential) of the two materials and the I coupled corrosion current density should be as small as possible.
2. The coupled corrosion potential of the couple combination should be significantly lower than the breakdown potential of the anodic component.
3. The repassivation properties of the anodic component of the couple should also be acceptable and these should be absence of a large hysteresis.

Cortada et al in 2000 investigated corrosion of five materials for implant suprastructues (cast-titanium, machined-titanium, gold alloy, silver-palladium alloy and chromium-nickel alloy), in vitro, the materials being galvanically coupled to a titanium implant. Various electrochemical parameters (E corr, icorr. Evans diagrams, polarization resistance and Tafel slopes) were analyzed. The microstructure of the different dental materials was observed before and after corrosion process by optical and electron microscopy. Besides, the metallic ions released in the saliva environment were quantified during the corrosion process by means of inductively coupled plasma-mass spectrometry technique (ICP-MS). The cast and machined titanium had the most passive current density at a given potential and chromium-nickel alloy and the most active critical current density values. The high gold content alloys have excellent resistance to corrosion, although this decreases when the gold content is lower in the alloy. The palladium alloy had a low critical current density due to the presence of gallium in this composition but a selective dissolution of copper rich phases was observed through energy dispersive X-ray analysis.

It is well known that the osseointegration of the commercially pure titanium (CP-Ti) dental implant is improved when the metal is shot blasted in order to increase its surface roughness. This roughness is colonized by bone, which improves implant fixation. However, shot blasting also changes the chemical composition of the implant surface because some shot particles remain adhered on the metal. The CP-Ti surfaces shot blasted with different materials and sizes of shot particles were tested in order to determine their topographical features (surface roughness, real surface area and the percentage of surface covered by the adhered shot particles) and electrochemical behavior (open circuit potential, electrochemical impedance spectroscopy and cyclic polarization). The results demonstrate that the increased surface area of the material because of the increasing surface roughness is not the only cause for the differences found in the electrochemical behavior and corrosion resistance of the blasted CP-Ti. Among other possible causes, those differences may be attributed to the compressive residual surface stresses induced by shot blasting.

Silverstein LH, Kurtzman GM in 2006 reported that oral hygiene maintenance is most important in implant long-term success. When dental implants were first introduced, the emphasis for long-term success was on the surgical phase of treatment. Subsequently, the emphasis changed from a focus on the surgical technique to proper fixture placement, which would be dictated by the prosthetic and aesthetic needs of each patient. In more recent years, implant maintenance and effective patient home care have been emphasized as two critical factors for long-term success of dental implants.

Christensen GJ in 2006 re-evaluated the importance approval and continuing observation of smaller diameter mini implants in situations in which standard sized implants (approximately 3.75 mm) could not be used without grafting. The result has been more patients who have been served successfully at reduced cost with minimized pain and trauma, patients who could not have been treated with implants otherwise.

Trakas T et al in 2006 reviewed a comparison between different attachment systems used to retain and support maxillary and mandibular overdentures in completely edentulous patients. The following factors were considered essential for successful outcome and good long-term prognosis of the prosthesis.

(i) Implant survival rate (ii) Marginal bone loss (iii) Soft tissue complications (iv) Retention (v) Stress distribution (vi) Space requirements (vii) Maintenance complications and (viii) Patient satisfaction.

Das Neves FD et al in 2006 studied to consider the therapeutic decision whether to use advanced surgery or short implants based on data concerning the use of these implants found in follow-up studies. The data was collected from articles published between 1980 and 2004. The analysis revealed that among the risk factors, poor bone quality in association with short implants seemed to be relevant to failure. The use of implants 4 mm in diameter appeared to minimize failure in these situations. The 3.75 × 7 m implant presented the highest failure rate. Thus it was concluded that short implants should be considered as an alternative to advanced bone augmentation surgeries. Since surgeries can involve higher morbidity, required extended clinical periods and involve higher costs to the patients.

Tortamano P et al in 2006 evaluated the survival and success of implants after immediate loading. A new method for to immediately load implants in edentulous patients was presented. Nine patients received 4 implants each resin metal prostheses were installed less than 48 hours after implant placement. Follow-up studies were done 6, 12, 24 months after surgery. None of them failed. It was proved that implants can be immediately loaded without jeopardizing osseointegration, if parameters are met, such as suitable bone quality and quantity, lack of unfavorable systemic and psychological factors, lack of parafunctional habits, strict maintenance of prosthetic requirement minimization of micromotion and use of an appropriate surgical protocol.

Implants Glossary

- **Abutment** Transmucosal abutment (TMA), links the implant body to the mouth. May be pre-manufactured or custom formed.
- **Alloplastic** Related to implantation of an inert foreign body.
- **Ankylosis** A condition of joint or tooth immobility resulting from oral pathology, surgery or direct contact with bone.
- **Anodization** An oxidation process in which a film is produced on the surface of a metal by electrolyte treatment at anode.
- **Bioacceptance** Ability to be tolerated in a biological environment in spite of adverse effects.
- **Bioactive** Capable of promoting the formation of hydroxyapatite and bonding to bone.
- **Biocompatibility** Ability of material to elicit an appropriate biological response in a given application of body.
- **Biointegration** Process in which bone or other living tissue becomes integrated with an implanted material with no intervening space.
- **Ceradapt abutment** It is developed to simplify the implant restorative procedures. This is accomplished with tooth colored, a precision milled, single ceramic component which can be prepared, customized and adapted to variation in implant position as well as peri-implant soft tissue anatomy.
- **Cover screw** Prevents bone ingress in implant head.
- **Diagnostic stent** It is fabricated with acrylic material planned implant site and filled with radiopaque material (for CT scan) and steel sphere (placed for OPG). It is worn by patient during radiographic examination.
- **Endosteal implant** A device that is placed into the alveolar and/or basal bone of the mandible or maxilla,which transects only one cortical plate.
- **Epithelial implant** A device placed within the oral mucosa.
- **Estheticone abutment** Estheticone abutment is designed to be used in multiple implant situations. If the traditional abutment might cause esthetic compromise with metal

display. It is designed to allow esthetic veneering material to be placed subgingivally.

- **Healing caps** Temporary covers for abutments.
- **Immediate implant** When implants are inserted at the time of extraction. They are called immediate implants.
- **Immediate loading implants** When the prosthesis is given immediately after the implant placement. The prosthesis is kept out of occlusion in such type of implants.
- **Implant analog** It is a replica of the implant screw, which simulates the position of the implant in the jaw, and attached with the impression post. This assembly of post and analog in the impression are poured in dental stone, so that the analog housed itself in the same way as it is housed in the patient's jaw.
- **Implantation** A process of grafting or inserting a material such as inert foreign body (alloplast) or tissue within the body.
- **Impression coping** Components of implant in any system used to transfer the location of the implant body or abutment to a dental cast.
- **Impression post/transfer** It is an accessory attached to the implant screw in the patient's mouth before making the impression.
- **Ion implantation** A process of altering the surface of metal with desirable ionic species.
- **Laboratory analogue** A base metal replica of the implant, or a pre-manufactured abutment.
- **Microimplant** Implants smaller in dimension used as anchorage in orthodontic treatment.
- **One-stage/two-stage implant** When implant insertion and fabrication of prosthesis are performed at the same time. This is called one-stage implant. But when the prosthesis is fabricated after 3-4 months of the insertion of the implant after re-opening the site, that is called two-stage implants.
- **Osseoinductive** Ability to promote bone formation through a mechanism that induces the differentiation of osteoblasts.
- **Osseointegration** Process in which living bony tissue forms to within the implant surface without any intervening fibrous connective tissue.

- **Passivation** Process of transforming a chemically active surface of metal to less active surface.
- **Procera abutment** Abutment can be designed by a computer and forwarded to a manufacturing facility by modem where abutment is machined to the exact specification developed in designing process. It is returned to the network laboratory for finalization of implant restoration by the dental technician.
- **Replantation** Reinsertion of a tooth back into its jaw socket soon after intentional extraction or accidental removal.
- **Sub-periosteal implant** A dental device that is placed beneath periosteum and overlies cortical bone.
- **Surgical template** Diagnostic stent converted into surgical stent by removing acrylic in implant placement area and placed during surgical procedure to guide implant position.
- **Temporary components** Pre-manufactured components of any dental implant system, used to make temporary crowns and bridges for fitting on dental implants and abutments.
- **Texturing** Process of increasing surface roughness of the area to which bone can bond.
- **Titanium** It is the best implant material, which is plasma sprayed/coated with thin layer of tri-calcium phosphate of hydroxyapatite.
- **Titanium alloys (Ti-6Al-4V)** Titanium with approximately 6 percent aluminum and 4 percent vanadium, most commonly used implant material.
- **Toxicity** Ability of material to cause cell or tissue death.
- **Transosteal implant** A device that penetrates both cortical plates and thickness of the alveolar bone.

Bibliography

1. Abe Y, Hiasa K, Takeuchi M, Yoshida X, Suzuki K, Abagawa Y. New surface modification of titanium implant with phosphoamino acid. Dent Mater J 2005; 24(4):536-40.

2. Adams PB. Anchoring means for false teeth US patent No. 2, 112, 007, March 22, 1938.

3. Al Hashimi I. The management of Sjögren's syndrome in dental practice. J Am Dent Assoc 2001;132:1409-17.

4. Al Hashimi I, Drinnan AJ, Uthman AA, Wright JR, Levine MJ. Oral amyloidosis: Two unusual case presentations. Oral Surg Oral Med Oral Pathol 1987; 63:586-91.

5. Albert D Gukes, Mark S Scurria, Tonya S King, George R Mccathy, Jaime S Brahim. Prospective clinical trial of dental implants in persons with ectodermal dysplasia. J Prosthet Dent 2002;88:21-5.

6. Albrektsson T, Blomberg S, Branemark A, et al. Edentulousness: An oral handicap. Patient reactions to treatment with jawbone-anchored prosthesis. J Oral Rehab 1987;14:503-11.

7. Albrektsson T, Zarb GA, Worthington P, et al. The long-term efficacy of currently used dental implants: A review and proposed criteria for success. Int J Oral Maxillofac Impl 1986;1:1-25.

8. Ales G Celar, Gerlinde Durstberger and Konstanin Zauza. Use of an individual traction prosthesis and distraction osteogenesis to reposition osseointegrated implants in a juvenile with ectodermal dysplasia: A clinical report. J Prosthet Dent 2002;87:145-8.

9. Ameen Kharaisat. Influence of occlusal forces on stress distribution. JPD 2004;91:319-25.

10. American Dental Association. Acceptance program for endosseous implants: Council of Dental Materials, Instruments and Equipment, Chicago, July 1993-97; American Dental Association.

11. Aparicio C, Gil FJ, Fonseca C, Barbosa M, Planell JA. Corrosion behavior of commercially pure titanium shot blasted with different materials and sizes of shot particles for dental implant applications. Biomaterials. 2003;24(2):263-73.

12. Arillo A, Melodia F, Frache R. Reduction of hexavalent chromium by mitochondria: Methodological implications and possible mechanisms. Ecotoxicol Environ Safety 1987;14:164-77.

13. Artzi Z, et al. Mucosal considerations for osseointegrated implants. JPD 1993;70:421-32.

14. Arvidson K, Bystedt H, Frykholm A, von Konow L, Lothigius E. A 3-year clinical study of Astra dental implants in the treatment of edentulous mandibles. Int J Oral Maxillofac Implants 1992;7:321-29.

15. Atkinson JC, Fox PC. Sjögren's syndrome: Oral and dental considerations. J Am Dent Assoc 1993;124:74-82, 84.

16. August M, Chung K, Chang Y, Glowacki J. Influence of estrogen status on endosseous implant osseointegration. J Oral Maxillofac Surg 2001;59:1285-9.

17. Babbush CA. Endosseous bladevent implants: A research review. J Oral Surg 1972;30:168-75.

18. Babbush CA. Personal communication, 1989 cited by Block, in implants in dentistry.

19. Bain CA, Moy PK. The association between the failure of dental implants and cigarette smoking. Int J Oral Maxillofac Implants 1993;8:609-15.

20. Balshi TJ, Wolfinger GJ. Dental implants in the diabetic patient: A retrospective study. Implant Dent 1999;8:355-9.

21. Beikler T, Flemmig TF. Antimicrobials in implant dentistry. In: Antibiotic and antimicrobial use in dental practice. Newman M, van Winkelhoff A (Eds). Chicago: Quintessence 2001;195-211.

22. Bergendal B, Bergendal T, Hallonsten AL, Koch G, Kurol J, Kvint S. A multidisciplinary approach to oral rehabilitation with osseointegrated implants in children and adolescents with multiple aplasia. Eur J Orthod 1996;18:119-29.

23. Bergendal T, Eckerdal O, Hallonsten AL, Koch G, Kurol J, Kvint S. Osseointegrated implants in the oral habilitation of a boy with ectodermal dysplasia: A case report. Int Dent J 1991;41:149-56.

24. Berglungh T, Lindhe J, Ericsson I, et al. The soft tissue

barrier at implants and teeth. Clin Oral Impl Res 1991;2:81-90.

25. Bianco PD, Ducheyne P, Cuckler JM. Biomaterials 1937;1996:17.

26. Binon P. Implants and components: Entering a new millennium. Int J Oral Maxillofac Implants 2000;15(1): 76-93.

27. Binon PP, Fowler CN. Implant-supported fixed prosthesis of four osseointegrated oral implant systems. J Mat Sci Mater Med 1993;8:54-60.

28. Blanchaert RH. Implants in the medically challenged patient. Dent Clin North Am 1998;42:35-45.

29. Block MS, Kent JN. Factors associated with soft and hard tissue compromise of endosseous implants. J Oral Maxillofac Surg 1990;48:1153-60.

30. Block PL, Wiley MG. Correction of alveolar ridge deformities with titanium implants. J Prosthet Dent 1988;60(R):221-5.

31. Blomberg S, Lundquist S. Psychological reaction to edentulousness and treatment with jawbone anchored bridges. J Prosthet Dent 1983;50:262-70.

32. Blomqvist JE, Alberius P, Isaksson S, Linde A, Hansson BG. Factors in implant integration failure after bone grafting: An osteometric and endocrinologic matched analysis. Int J Oral Maxillofac Surg 1996;25:63-8.

33. Bothe RT, Beaton LE, Davenport HA. Reaction of bone to multiple metallic implants. Surg Gynecol Obstet 1940; 71:598-602, cited by Carl E Misch.

34. Boutsi EA, Paikos S, Dafni UG, Moutsopoulos HM, Skopouli FN. Dental and periodontal status of Sjögren's syndrome. J Clin Periodontol 2000;27:231-5.

35. Brain H Williams, Kent T Ochiai, Satoru Hojo, Russel Nishimura, Angelo A. Caputo: Retention of maxillary implant overdenture bars of different designs. J Prosthet Dent 2001;86:603-7.

36. Branemark PI, Adell R, Breine U, Hansson BO, Lindstrom J, Ohlsson A. Intraosseous anchorage of dental prosthesis: Experimental Studies. Scand J Plas Reconst Surg 1969;3:81-100.

37. Branemark PI, Hansson BO, Adell R, Breine U, Lindstrom J, Halloeno, et al. Osseointegrated implants

in the treatment of the edentulous jaw: Experience from a 10-year period. Scand J Plast Reconstr Surg Suppl 1997;16:1-132.

38. Breeding LC, Dixon DL, Schmitt S. The effect of simulated function on the retention of bar clip retained removal prostheses. J Prosthet Dent 1996;75:570-3.

39. Budtz-Jørgensen E. The significance of Candida albicans in denture stomatitis. Scand J Dent Res 1974; 82:151-90.

40. Budtz-Jørgensen E, Lombardi T. Antifungal therapy in the oral cavity. Periodontol 1996;2000;10:89-106.

41. Bullon P, Pascual A, Fernandez-Novoa MC, Borobio MV, Muniain MA, Camacho F. Late onset Papillon-Lefévre syndrome? A chromosomic, neutrophil function and microbiological study. J Clin Periodontol 1993;20:662-67.

42. Burke JF. The effective period of preventive antibiotic action in experimental incisions and dermal lesions. Surgery 1961;124:268-76.

43. Cann CE, Genant HK, Kolb FO, Ettinger B. Quantitative computed tomography for prediction of vertebral fracture risk. Bone 1985;6:1-7.

44. Carl Mish (contemporary implant dentistry, new 2nd edition.

45. Carlo E Poggio, Antonnio Salvato. Implant repositioning for esthetic reasons: A clinical report. J Prosthet Dent 2001;86:126-9.

46. Carmine, et al. Spreading of epithelial cells on machined and sand blasted surfaces. Journal of Periodontology 2003;74:289-95.

47. Chotiros Kuphasuk, Yoshiki Oshida, Carl J Andres, Suteera T Hovijitra, Martin T Barco, David T Brown. Electrochemical corrosion of titanium and titanium-based alloys. J Prosthet Dent 2001;85:195-202.

48. Christensen GJ. The mini-implant has arrived. J Am Den Assoc 2006;137(3):387-90.

49. Clarke A. Hypohidrotic ectodermal dysplasia. J Med Genet 1987;24:659-63.

50. Cohen MD, Kargacin B, Klein CB, Costa M. Mechanisms of Chromium carcinogenicity and toxicity. Crit Rev Toxicol 1993;23:255-81.

51. Cooper LF. Systemic effectors of alveolar bone mass and implications in dental therapy. Periodontol 2000;23:103-9.

52. Cortada M, Giner L, Costa S, Gil FJ, Rodriguez D, Planell JA. Galvanic Corrosion behavior of titanium implants coupled to dental alloys. J Mater Sci Mater Med 2000;11 (5):287-93.

53. Cortada M, Giner L, Costa S, Gil FJ, Rodriguez D, Planell JA. Metallic ion release in different metal super-structures. Biomed Mater Eng 1997;7(3):213-20.

54. Cranin AN. Endosteal implants in a patient with corticosteroid dependence. J Oral Implantol 1991;17:414-7.

55. Cranin AN, Silverbrand H, Sher J, Satler N. The requirements and clinical performance of dental implants In: Smita DS, Williams DF (Eds), Biocompatibility of dental materials Vol 5, Chapter 10. CRC Press: Boca Raton F1 1982.

56. Cronin RJ, Oesterle LJ. Implant use in growing patients. Treatment planning concerns. Dent Clin North Am 1998;42:1-34.

57. Curator, Peabody Museum, Harvard University. Personal Communication, 1994; cited by MS Block in implants in dentistry.

58. Curtis M Becker, David A Kaiser, John D Jones. Guidelines for splinting implants. J Prosthet Dent 2000;84:210-4.

59. Dahlin, et al. Generation of new bone around titanium implants using a membrane techniques. Int Oral and Max Surg 1989;4:19-25.

60. Dajani AS, Taubert KA, Wilson W, Bolger AF, Bayer A, Ferrieri P, et al. Prevention of bacterial endocarditis: Recommendations by the American Heart Association. Clin Infect Dis 1997;25:1448-58.

61. Dalton JE. Effects of surgical fit and hydroxyapatite coating on the mechanical and biological response to porous implants. Master's thesis, Tulane University New Orleans, 1991.

62. Dao TT, Anderson JD, Zarb GA. Is osteoporosis a risk factor for osseointegration of dental implants? Int J Oral Maxillofac Implants 1993;8:137-44.

63. Darnell JA, Saunders MJ. Oral manifestations of the diabetic patient. TX Dent J 1990;107:23-7.

64. Davarpanah M, Moon JW, Yang LR, Celletti R, Martinez H. Dental implants in the oral rehabilitation of a teenager with hypohidrotic ectodermal dysplasia: Report of a case. Int J Oral Maxillofac Implants 1997;12:252-8.

65. Debetto P, Luciani S. Toxic effect of chromium on cellular metabolism Sci Total Environ 1988;71:365-77.

66. Delamaire M, Maugendre D, Moreno M, Le Goff MC, Allannic H, Genetet B. Impaired leukocyte functions in diabetic patients. Diabet Med 1997;14:29-34.

67. Dent CD, Olson JW, Farish SE, Bellome J, Casino AJ, Morris HF, et al. The influence of preoperative antibiotics on success of endosseous implants up to and including stage II surgery: A study of 2,641 implants. J Oral Maxillofac Surg 1997;55:19-24.

68. Devorah Schwatz, et al. The clinical effectiveness of implants placed immediately into fresh extraction sites of molar teeth. JP 2000;71:839-44.

69. Dhanrajani PJ, Jiffry AO. Management of ectodermal dysplasia: A literature review. Dent Update 1998;25:73-5.

70. Dietschi D, Schatz JP. Current restorative modalities for young patients with missing anterior teeth. Quintessence Int 1997;28:231-40.

71. Dov M. Almog, Rodolfo Sanchez. Correlation between planned prosthetic and residual bone trajectories in dental implants. J Prosthet Dent 1999;81:562-7.

72. Drosos AA, Constantopoulos SH, Psychos D, Stefanou D, Papadimitriou CS, Moutsopoulos HM. The forgotten cause of sicca complex; sarcoidosis. J Rheumatol 1989;16:1548-51.

73. Duarte PM, Nogueira Filho GR, Sallum EA, de Toledo S, Sallum AW, Nociti Junior FH. The effect of an immunosuppressive therapy and its withdrawal on bone healing around titanium implants. A histometric study in rabbits. J Periodontol 2001;72:1391-7.

74. Eder A, Watzek G. Treatment of a patient with severe osteoporosis and chronic polyarthritis with fixed implant-supported prosthesis: A case report. Int J Oral Maxillofac Implants 1999;14:587-90.

75. Edmond Bedrossian and Lambert J Stumpel. Immediate stabilization at stage II of zygomatic implants: Rationale and technique. J Prosthet Dent 2001;86:10-4.

76. Ekstrand K, Thomsson M. Ectodermal dysplasia with partial anodontia: Prosthetic treatment with implant fixed prosthesis. ASDC J Dent Child 1988;55:282-4.

77. el Askary AS, Meffert RM, Griffin T. Why do dental implants fail? Part I. Implant Dent 1999;8:173-85.

78. Elders PJ, Netelenbos JC, Lips P, van Ginkel FC, van der Stelt PF. Accelerated vertebral bone loss in relation to the menopause: A cross-sectional study on lumbar bone density in 286 women of 46 to 55 years of age. Bone Miner 1988;5:11-9.

79. Engleman M. Clinical decision and treatment planning in osseointegration. Coral Stream (IL): Quintessence Publishing Co Inc 1996;187-92.

80. Escobar V, Epker BN. Alveolar bone growth in response to endosteal implants in two patients with ectodermal dysplasia. Int J Oral Maxillofac Surg 1998;27:445-7.

81. Esposito M, Hirsch JM, Lekholm U, Thomson P. Biological factors contributing to failures of osseo-integrated oral implants (II): Etiopathogenesis. Eur J Oral Sci 1998;106:721-64.

82. Esposito M, Hirsch JM, Lekholm U, Thomson P. Failure patterns of four osseointegrated oral implant systems. J Mat Sci Mater Med 1997;8:843-7.

83. Falk H, Laurell, Lundgren D. Occlusal force pattern in dentitions with mandibular implant-supported fixed cantilever prostheses occluded with complete dentures. Int J Oral Maxillofac Implants 1989;4:55-62.

84. Farah CS, Ashman RB, Challacombe SJ. Oral candidosis. Clin Dermatol 2000;18:553-62.

85. Fiorellini JP, Chen PK, Nevins M, Nevins ML. A retrospective study of dental implants in diabetic patients. Int J Periodont Rest Dent 2000;20:366-73.

86. Fiorellini JP, Nevins ML, Norkin A, Weber HP, Karimbux NY. The effect of insulin therapy on osseointegration in a diabetic rat model. Clin Oral Implants Res 1999;10:362-8.

87. Fischer K, Stenberg T. Three-year data from a randomized, controlled study of early loading of single

stage dental implants supporting maxillary full-arch prosthesis. Int J Oral Maxillofac Implants. March-April 2006;21(2):245-52.

88. Fox PC. Acquired salivary dysfunction. Drugs and radiation. Ann NY Acad Sci 1998;842:132-7.

89. Friberg B. Treatment with dental implants in patients with severe osteoporosis: A case report. Int J Periodont Rest Dent 1994;14:348-53.

90. Fu E, Hsieh YD, Shen EC, Nieh S, Mao TK, Chiang CY. Cyclosporin-induced gingival overgrowth at the newly formed edentulous ridge in rats: A morphological and histometric evaluation. J Periodontol 2001;72:889-94.

91. Fugazzotto PA, Gulbransen HJ, Wheeler SL, Lindsay JA. The use of IMZ osseointegrated implants in partially and completely edentulous patients: Success and failure rates of 2,023 implant cylinders up to 60+ months in function. Int J Oral Maxillofac Implants 1993;8:617-21.

92. Fujimoto T, Niimi A, Nakai H, Ueda M. Osseointegrated implants in a patient with osteoporosis: A case report. Int J Oral Maxillofac Implants 1996;11:539-42.

93. Fujimoto T, Niimi A, Sawai T, Ueda M. Effects of steroid-induced osteoporosis on osseointegration of titanium implants. Int J Oral Maxillofac Implants 1998;13:183-9.

94. Gamborena JI, Hazelton LR, Na Budalung D, Brudvik J. Retention of ERA direct overdenture attachments before and after fatigue loading. Int J Prosthodont 1997;10:123-30.

95. Gammage DD, Bowman AE, Meffert RM, et al. A histologic and scanning electron micrographic comparison of osseous interface in loaded IMZ and integral implants. Int J Periodont 1990;10:125-135.

96. Garg A. Pharmacological agents used in implant dentistry. Implant Soc 1992;3:1,5-7,16.

97. Garnero P, Delmas PD. Osteoporosis. Endocrinol Metab Clin North Am 1997;26:913-36.

98. Geerlings SE, Hoepelman AI. Immune dysfunction in patients with diabetes mellitus (DM). FEMS Immunol Med Microbiol 1999;26:259-65.

99. Geis GJ, Weber JG, Sauer KH. *In vitro* substance loss due to galvanic corrosion in titanium implant/Ni-Cr superconstruction systems. Int J Oral Maxillofac Imp 1994;9:449-54.

100. Gerritsen M, Lutterman JA, Jansen JA. Wound healing around bone-anchored percutaneous devices in experimental diabetes mellitus. J Biomed Mater Res 2000;53:702-9.

101. Gift and Newman. How older adults use oral health care services: Results of a national health interview surgery. J Am Dent Assoc 1993;124:89-93.

102. Glaser DL, Kaplan FS. Osteoporosis. Definition and clinical presentation. Spine 1997;22:12S-16S.

103. Goldberg NI, Gershkoff A. The implant lower denture. Dent Diag 1949;55:490-3.

104. Gonzales TS, Coleman GC. Periodontal manifestations of collagen vascular disorders. Periodontol 1999;2000; 21:94-105.

105. Gottlander M, Johansson CB, Albrektsson T. Short and long-term studies with a plasma sprayed calcium phosphate-coated implant. Clin Oral Implants Res 1997;8:345-51.

106. Granstrom, et al. Titanium implants in irradiated tissue benefits from hyperbaric oxygen. Int J of Oral and Max Surgery 1992;7:15-25.

107. Green NT. Fracture of Dental Implants: Literature Review and report of a case. Imp Dent 2002;137:143.

108. Greenfield EJ. Implantation of artificial crowns and bridge abutments. Dent Cosmos 1913; 55:304-430, cited by Carl E Misch.

109. Grisius MM. Salivary gland dysfunction: A review of systemic therapies. Oral Surg Oral Med Oral Pathol Oral Radiol Endod 2001;92:156-62.

110. Groessner-Schreiber B, Nubert A, Muller WD, Hopp M, Grepentrog M, Lange KP. Fibroblast growth on surface modified dental implants: An *in vitro* study. J Biomed Mater Res 2003;64A(4):591-9.

111. Grosgogeat B, Reclaru L, Lissac M, Dalard F. Measurement and evaluation of galvanic corrosion between titanium/Ti-6Al-4V implants and dental alloys by

electrochemical techniques and auger spectrometry. Biomaterials 1999;20:933-41.

112. Guchelaar HJ, Vermes A, Meerwaldt JH. Radiation-induced xerostomia: Pathophysiology, clinical course and supportive treatment. Support Care Cancer 1997;5:281-8.

113. Guckes AD, Brahim JS, McCarthy GR, Rudy SF, Cooper LF. Using endosseous dental implants for patients with ectodermal dysplasia. J Am Dent Assoc 1991;122:59-62

114. Guckes AD, McCarthy GR, Brahim J. Use of endosseous implants in a 3-year-old child with ectodermal dysplasia: Case report and 5-year follow-up. Pediatr Dent 1997;19:282-5.

115. Guckes AD, Roberts MW, McCarthy GR. Pattern of permanent teeth present in individuals with ectodermal dysplasia and severe hypodontia suggests treatment with dental implants. Pediatr Dent 1998;20:278-80.

116. Guera, et al. Tissue supported implant overdentures. Imp Dent 1992;1:69-77.

117. Guo CY, Johnson A, Locke TJ, Eastell R. Mechanisms of bone loss after cardiac transplantation. Bone 1998;22:267-71.

118. Harel Simon. Use of transitional implants to support a surgical guide: Enhancing accuracy of implant placement. J Prosthet Dent 2002;87:229-32.

119. Harris D. Advanced surgical procedures: Bone augmentation. Dent Update 1997;24:332-7.

120. Harris LM. An artifical crown on a leaden root, Dent Cosmos 1887;55:433, cited by Carl E. Misch.

121. Harris MI, Flegal KM, Cowie CC, Eberhardt MS, Goldstein DE, Little RR, et al. Prevalence of diabetes, impaired fasting glucose, and impaired glucose tolerance in US adults. The Third National Health and Nutrition Examination Survey, 1988-1994. Diabetes Care 1998;21:518-24.

122. Hartman GA. Effect of initial implant position on magnitude and crestal bone remodeling. Journal of periodontology 2004.

123. Heersche JN, Bellows CG, Ishida Y. The decrease in bone mass associated with aging and menopause. J Prosthet Dent 1998;79:14-6.

124. Heimke G, Kolbe RJ, Latour Jr RA. The engineering background of the concept of isoelastic implants. J Mat Sci Mater Med 1992;3:204-11.

125. Hermann JS, Buser D. Guided bone regeneration for dental implants. Curr Opin Periodontol 1996;3:168-77.

126. Hildebolt CF. Osteoporosis and oral bone loss. Dentomaxillofac Radiol 1997;26:3-15.

127. Hille GH. Titanium for surgical implants. J Mat 1966; 1:373-83.

128. Hillenburg KL, Kosinski TF, Mentag PJ. Control of peri-implant inflammation. Pract Periodont Aesthet Dent 1991;3:11-6.

129. Horasawa N, Takahashi S, Marekb M. Galvanic interaction between titanium and gallium alloy or dental amalgam. Dent Mater 1999;15(5):318-22.

130. Ibanez, et al. Performance of acid-etched surface external hex implants in relation to one- and two-stage procedure. Journal of Periodontology 2003;74:1575-81.

131. Indira G Sahiwal, Ronald D Woody, Byron W Benson, Guillermo E Guillen. Radiographic identification of non-threaded endosseous dental implants. J Prosthet Dent 2002;87:552-62.

132. Ioannidou. Osteotome sinus floor elevation and simultaneous non-submerged implant placement: Case report and review. JP 2000;71:1613-9.

133. Iwabuchi Y, Katagiri M, Masuhara T. Salivary secretion and histopathological effects after single administration of the muscarinic agonist SNI-2011 in MRL/lpr mice. Arch Int Pharmacodyn Ther 1994;328:315-25.

134. Iwabuchi Y, Masuhara T. Sialogogic activities of SNI-2011 compared with those of pilocarpine and McN-A-343 in rat salivary glands: Identification of a potential therapeutic agent for treatment of Sjögren's syndrome. Gen Pharmacol 1994;25:123-9.

135. Iyama S, Takeshita F, Ayukawa Y, Kido MA, Suetsugu T, Tanaka T. A study of the regional distribution of

bone formed around hydroxyapatite implants in the tibiae of streptozotocin-induced diabetic rats using multiple fluorescent labeling and confocal laser scanning microscopy. J Periodontol 1997;68:1169-75.

136. Jacobs JJ, Gilbert JL, Urbani RM. Corrosion of Metal Orhopedic Implants. J Bone Joint Surg 1988;80:1-2.

137. Jan Lindhe. Osseointegration historic background current concepts, clinical periodontology and implant dentistry pp, 808-13.

138. Jeffcoat MK, Lewis CE, Reddy MS, Wang CY, Redford M. Post-menopausal bone loss and its relationship to oral bone loss. Periodontol 2000;23:94-102.

139. Jian-Ping Geng, Keson BC Tom, Gui Rong Liu. Application of finite element analysis in implant dentistry: A review of literature. J Prosthet Dent 2001;85:585-98.

140. Johansson Bl, Bergman B. Corrosion of titanium and amalgam couples: Effect of fluoride, area size, surface preparation and fabrication procedures. Dent Mater 1995;1:41-6.

141. Johnson BW. HA-coated dental implants: Long-term consequences. J CA Dent Assoc 1992;20:33-41.

142. Jovanovic SA. Diagnosis and treatment of peri-implant disease. Curr Opin Periodontol 1994;2:194-204.

143. Judith L Gartner, Kazuhiko Mushimoto, Hans Peter Weber, Ichiro Nishimura. Effect of osseointegrated implants on the coordination of masticatory muscles: A pilot study. J Prosthet Dent 2000;84:185-93.

144. Kahan BD. Cyclosporine. N Engl J Med 1989;321:1725-38.

145. Kalpiedis, et al. Review of hemorrhage incidence in case of implant placement in anterior mandible. Journal of periodontology 2004;75:631-45.

146. Kapur KK, Garrett NR, Hamada MO, Roumanas ED, Freymiller E, Han T, et al. A randomized clinical trial comparing the efficacy of mandibular implant-supported overdentures and conventional dentures in diabetic patients. Part I: Methodology and clinical outcomes. J Prosthet Dent 1998;79:555-69.

147. Kearns G, Sharma A, Perrott D, Schmidt B, Kaban L, Vargervik K. Placement of endosseous implants in children and adolescents with hereditary ectodermal dysplasia. Oral Surg Oral Med Oral Pathol Oral Radiol Endod 1999;88:5-10.

148. Kirsch A, Ackermann KL. The IMZ osseointegrated implant system. Dent Clin of North Am 1989;33:733-91.

149. Kitichai Rungcharassaeng, Jaime L. Lozada, Joseph YK Khan, Jay S Kim, Wayne V Campagni and Carlos A. Munoz. Peri-implant tissue response of immediately loaded, threaded, HA-coated implants: 1-year results. J Prosthet Dent 2002;87:173-81.

150. Klokkevold PR. Periodontal medicine: Assessment of risk factors for disease. J CA Dent Assoc 1999;27:135-42.

151. Kordossis T, Paikos S, Aroni K, Kitsanta P, Dimitrakopoulos A, Kavouklis E, et al. Prevalence of Sjögren's-like syndrome in a cohort of HIV-1-positive patients: Descriptive pathology and immunopathology. Br J Rheumatol 1998;37:691-5.

152. Krane SM, Holick MF. Metabolic bone diseases. In: Principles of internal medicine. Wilson JD, Braunwald EB, Isselbacher KJ, Petersdorf RG, Martin JB, Fauci AS, et al (Eds). New York: McGraw-Hill, 1991;1921-32.

153. Kraut RA. Dental implants for children: Creating smiles for children without teeth. Pract Periodont Aesthet Dent 1996;8:909-13.

154. Kribbs PJ. Comparison of mandibular bone in normal and osteoporotic women. J Prosthet Dent 1990;63:218-22.

155. Kribbs PJ, Chesnut CH III, Ott SM, Kilcoyne RF. Relationships between mandibular and skeletal bone in an osteoporotic population. J Prosthet Dent 1989;62:703-7.

156. Krolner B, Nielson SP. Clinical application of dual photon absorptiometry of the lumbar vertebrae. In: Non-invasive bone measurements: Methodological problems. Dequeker J, Johnston CC (Eds). Oxford: IRL Press, 1982;201-5.

157. Lang, et al. Lingualized integration: Tooth moulds and an occlusal scheme for edentulous implant patients. Impt Dent 1992;1:204-11.

158. Lang NP, Mombelli A, Brägger U, Hammerle CH. Monitoring disease around dental implants during supportive periodontal treatment. Periodontol 1996;2000;12:60-8.

159. Larkin JG, Frier BM, Ireland JT. Diabetes mellitus and infection. Postgrad Med J 1985;61:233-7.

160. Laster Z, Weisberg A, Gershonovitch S and Baruch D. A new tricortical implant. Refant Hapeh Vehashinayim 2003;20(3):89-95,105.

161. Ledermann PD, Schroeder A, Sutter F. Single tooth replacement with the aid of the ITI (International Team Fur Implantologie) type F hollow cylinder implant (late implant). SSO Schweiz Monatsschr Zahnheilkd (German) 1982;92:1087-98.

162. Lee TC. History of dental implants in Cramin An (Ed.) Oral Implantology. Spring Field, III, Charles C Thomas, 1970, pp 3-5.

163. Lee YT and Welsch G. Youngs modulus and damping capacity of Ti-6Al-4V (Proc. of the conference), Ti Science and Technology, Plenum Press, 1984;1689-96.

164. Leinfelder KF, Lemons JE. Clinical restorative materials and Techniques. Ler and Febiger: Philadelphia 1998; 139-59.

165. Lemons J, Nahiella J. Biomaterials biocompatibility and peri-implant considerations. Dent Clin North Am 1986; 30:4.

166. Levin L, Schwartz-Arad D. The effect of cigarette smoking on dental implants and related surgery. Implant Dent 2005;14(4):357-61.

167. Lewis S, Beumer J 3rd, Hornburg W, Moy P. The "ULCA" abutment. Int J Oral Maxillofac Implants 1988;3: 183-9.

168. Linkow LI. The bladevent: A new dimensions in endosseous implantology. Dental Concepts, Spring; 1968.

169. Litsky AS, Spector M. 'Biomaterials' In: Simon SR (Ed.) Orthopedic basic science. Am Acad Orthop Surg 1994; 470-3.

170. Looker AC, Orwoll ES, Johnston CC, Lindsay RL, Wahner HW, Dunn WL, et al. Prevalence of low femoral bone density in older US adults from NHANES III. J Bone Miner Res 1997;12:1761-8.

171. Lord BJ. Maintenance procedures for the implant patient. Aust Prosthodont J 1995;9(Suppl):33-8.

172. Lucas LC, Lemons JD. Biodegradation of restorative metallic systems. Adv Dent Res 1992;6:32-7.

173. Lugero GG, de Falco Carpalo V, Guzzo ML, Konig B, Jorgetti V. Histomorphometric evaluation of titanium implants in osteoporotic rabbits. Implant Dent 2000; 9:303-9.

174. Lum LB, Beirne OR, Dillinges M, Curtis TA. Osseointegration of two types of implants in non-human primates. J Prosthet Dent 1988;60(6):700-5.

175. Lundgren D, Falk H, Laurel L. Influence of number and distribution of occlusal cantilever contacts on closing and chewing forces in dentitions with implant supported fixed prostheses occluding with complete dentures. Int J Oral Maxillofac Implants 1989;4:277-83.

176. Lundquist S, Haraldson T. Occlusal perception of thickness in patients with bridges on osseointegrated oral implants. Scand J Dent Res 1984;92:88.

177. MacFarlane TW, Mason DK. Changes in the oral flora in Sjögren's syndrome. J Clin Pathol 1974;27:416-9.

178. Maggiolo. Maneul de l'art dentaire (Manual of Dental art) Nancy, France, 1809, C. Le Seuer; Cited by Carl E Misch in Contemporary Implant Dentistry 1993 edition, Mosby Yearbook, Inc. St-Louis, USA.

179. Martin D Gross, Joseph Nissan, Rellusamuel. Stress distribution around maxillary implants in anatomic photoelastic models of varying geometry. Part I. J Prosthet Dent 2001;85:442-9.

180. Martin D Gross, Joseph Nissan. Stress distribution around maxillary implants in anatomic photoelastic models of varying geometry. Part II. J Prosthet Dent 2001;85:450-4.

181. Mats Kronstrom, Tor Widbom, Lisebtt E. Lofquist, Christer Henningson, Christin Wibdom and Tomas

Lundberg. Early functional loading of conical Branemark implants in the endentulous mandible: A 12 month follow-up clinical report. J Prosthet Dent 2003;89:335-40.

182. Mauro Cruz, Clovis Cruz Reis and Flavio de Treitas Mattos. Implant induced expansion of atrophic ridges for placement of implants. J Prosthet Dent 2001;85:377-81.

183. McCracken M, Lemons JE, Rahemtulla F, Prince CW, Feldman D. Bone response to titanium alloy implants placed in diabetic rats. Int J Oral Maxillofac Implants 2000;15:345-54.

184. McDonald JA, Dunstan CR, Dilworth P, Sherbon K, Sheil AG, Evans RA, et al. Bone loss after liver transplantation. Hepatology 1991;14:613-9.

185. Meffert RM. Maintenance and treatment of the ailing and failing implant. J IN Dent Assoc 1994;73:22-4.

186. Meffert RM. Periodontitis vs. peri-implantitis: The same disease? The same treatment? Crit Rev Oral Biol Med 1996;7:278-91.

187. Melton LJ. Epidemiology of spinal osteoporosis. Spine 1997;22:2S-11S.

188. Melvin JE. Saliva and dental diseases. Curr Opin Dent 1991;1:795-801.

189. Mericske-Stern R, Zarb GA. Overdentures: An alternative implant methodology for edentulous patients. Int J Prosthodont 1993;6:203-8.

190. Merritt K, Brown SA. Release of hexavalent chromium from corrosion of stainless steel and cobalt-chromium alloys. J Biomed Mater Res 1995;29:627-33.

191. Merritt K, Fedele CD, Brown SA. Chromium 6?? or 3?? release during corrosion; and *in vivo* distribution. Biomater Tissue Interf 1992;49-53.

192. Minsk L, Polson AM. Dental implant outcomes in postmenopausal women undergoing hormone replacement. Compend Contin Educ Dent 1998;19:859-862, 864.

193. Misch CE. Bone character: Second vital implant criterian, Dent Today June/July 1988;39-40.

194. Misch CE. Dental education. Meeting the demands of implant dentistry. J Am Dent Assoc 1990;121:334-8.

195. Mombelli A. Etiology, diagnosis, and treatment considerations in peri-implantitis. Curr Opin Periodontol 1997;4:127-36.

196. Mombelli A, Lang NP. Antimicrobial treatment of peri-implant infections. Clin Oral Implants Res 1992;3: 162-8.

197. Moore, et al. Retrospective study of severely atrophied mandibular cases treated with sub-periosteal implants. JPD 2004;92:145-50.

198. Mori H, Manabe M, Kurachi Y, Nagumo M. Osseo-integration of dental implants in rabbit bone with low mineral density. J Oral Maxillofac Surg 1997;55:351-61.

199. Morris HF, Ochi S, Winkler S. Implant survival in patients with type 2 diabetes: Placement to 36 months. Ann Periodontol 2000;5:157-65.

200. Murrah VA. Diabetes mellitus and associated oral manifestations: A review. J Oral Pathol 1985;14:271-81.

201. Mustafa K, Silva Lopez B, Hultenby K, Wennerberg A, Arvindson K. Attachment and proliferation of human oral fibroblasts to titanium surfaces blasted with TiO_2 particles. A scanning electron microscopic and histomorphometric analysis. Clin Oral Implants Res 1998;9(3):195-207.

202. Nadia M Taher, Abed S. Al Jabab. Galvanic corrosion behavior of implant superstructure dental alloys. Dental Materials 2003;19:54-9.

203. Najera MP, al Hashimi I, Plemons JM, Rivera-Hidalgo F, Rees TD, Haghighat N, et al. Prevalence of perio-dontal disease in patients with Sjögren's syndrome. Oral Surg Oral Med Oral Pathol Oral Radiol Endod 1997;83:453-7.

204. Nancy R Chaffee, Kevin Lowden, John C. Tiffee and Lyndon F Cooper. Periapical abscess formation and resolution adjacent to dental implants: A clinical report. J Prosthet Dent 2001;85:109-12.

205. Nasu M, Amano Y, Kurita A, Yosue T. Osseointegration in implant-embedded mandible in rats fed calcium-

deficient diet: A radiological study. Oral Dis 1998;4: 84-9.

206. Nemcovsky. Interproximal papillae reconstruction in maxillary implants. JP 2000;71:308-14.

207. Nevins ML, Karimbux NY, Weber HP, Giannobile WV, Fiorellini JP. Wound healing around endosseous implants in experimental diabetes. Int J Oral Maxillofac Implants 1998;13:620-9.

208. NHS Research and Development Centre of Evidence-Based Medicine (accessed: 08-2002). Levels of evidence. Web page: http://www.cebm.net.

209. Nicola U Zitzmann and Carlo P Marinello. Treatment plan for restoring the edentulous maxilla with implant supported restorations: Removable overdentures versus fixed partial denture design. J Prosthet Dent 1999;82:188-96.

210. Nikolai J Altard and George A Zarb. Implant prostho-dontic management of partially edentulous patients missing posterior teeth: The Toronto Experience. J Prosthet Dent 2003;89:352-9.

211. Nivot Gival, et al. Emergency tracheostomy following life-threatening hemorrhage. JP 2000;71:1893-5.

212. Norman and Cranin. Atlas of oral implantology. Trans osseous implants 2nd ed.

213. Oesterle LJ, Cronin RJ, Ranly DM. Maxillary implants and the growing patient. Int J Oral Maxillofac Implants 1993;8:377-87.

214. Oh KT, Kim KN. Electrochemical properties of superstructures galvanically coupled to a titanium implant. J Biomed Mater Res B Appl Biomater August 14, 2004;70(2):318-31.

215. Olmedo D, Fernadez MM, Guglidmotti MB, Cabrini RL. Macrophages related to dental implant failure. Imp Dent 2003;12:75-80.

216. Olson JW, Shernoff AF, Tarlow JL, Colwell JA, Scheetz JP, Bingham SF. Dental endosseous implant assessments in a type 2 diabetic population: A prospective study. Int J Oral Maxillofac Implants 2000;15:811-8.

217. Orsini G, Assenza B, Scarano A, Piattelli A. Surface analysis of machined versus sandblasted and acid-

etched titanium implants. Int J Oral Maxillofac Implants 2000;15(6):779-84.

218. Osial TA, Whiteside TL, Buckingham RB, Singh G, Barnes EL, Pierce JM, et al. Clinical and serologic study of Sjögren's syndrome in patients with progressive systemic sclerosis. Arthritis Rheum 1983;26:500-8.

219. Ozyvaci H. Radiotherapy and histomorphometric evaluation of maxillary sinus grafting with alloplastic graft materials. Journal Periodontology 2004;74:909-15.

220. Pallasch TJ. Antifungal and antiviral chemotherapy. Periodontol 2000;28:240-55.

221. Pan J, Shirota T, Ohno K, Michi K. Effect of ovariectomy on bone remodeling adjacent to hydroxyapatite-coated implants in the tibia of mature rats. J Oral Maxillofac Surg 2002;58:877-82.

222. Paolo Trisisi, et al. Bone to implant contact on machined and acid etched surfaces after 2 months of placement in human maxilla. Journal of Periodontology 2004; 74:945-56.

223. Paolo Vigolo, Andrea Givani. Clinical evaluation of single-tooth mini-implant restorations: A five-year retrospective study. J Prosthet Dent 2000;84:50-4.

224. Payne AG, Lownie JF, Van Der Linden WJ. Implant-supported prostheses in patients with Sjögren's syndrome: A clinical report on three patients. Int J Oral Maxillofac Implants 1997;12:679-85.

225. Payne JB, Reinhardt RA, Nummikoski PV, Patil KD. Longitudinal alveolar bone loss in post-menopausal osteoporotic/osteopenic women. Osteoporos Int 1999;10:34-40.

226. Percinoto C, Vieira AE, Barbieri CM, Melhado FL, Moreira KS. Use of dental implants in children: A literature review. Quintessence Int 2001;32:381-3.

227. Periklis Proussaefs and Jaime Lozada. Evaluation of two vitallium blade-form implants retrieved after 13-21 years of function: A clinical report. J Prosthet Dent 2002;87:412-5.

228. Periklis Proussaefs. Histologic evaluation of a threaded hydroxyapatite-coated root-form implant located at a

dehisced maxillary site and retrieved from a human subject. J Prosthet Dent 2002;87:140-4.

229. Perizzolo D, Lacefield WR, Brenette DM. Interaction between topography and coating in the formation of bone nodules in culture for hydroxyapatite and titanium coated micromachined surfaces. J Biomed Mater Res 2001;56(4):494-503.

230. Peter M Gronet, Gregory A, Waskewicz and Charles Richardson. Preformed acrylic cranial implants using fused deposition modeling: A clinical report. J Prosthet Dent 2003;90:429-33.

231. Peterson LJ. Antibiotic prophylaxis against wound infections in oral and maxillofacial surgery. J Oral Maxillofac Surg 1990;48:617-20.

232. Petropoulus VC, Smith W, Kousvelari E. Comparison of retention and release periods for implant overdenture attachments. Int J Oral Maxillofac Implants 1997;12: 176-85.

233. Pilliar RM, Deporter DA, Watson PA, et al. Dental implant design: Effect on bone remodeling. J Biomed Mat Res 1991;25:467-83.

234. Pinheiro M, Freire-Maia N. Ectodermal dysplasias: A clinical classification and a causal review. Am J Med Genet 1994;53:153-62.

235. Pinheiro M, Freire-Maia N. Ectodermal dysplasias. In: Inherited skin disorders: The genodermatoses. Harper J (Ed.). Oxford: Butterworth-Heinemann, 1996;126-44.

236. Porter JA, Von Fraunhofer JA. Success of failure of dental implants? A literature review with treatment considerations. Gen Dent 2005;53(6):423-32; Quiz 433, 446.

237. Pourbaix M. Electrochemical corrosion of metallic biomaterials. Biomaterials 1984;5(3):122-34.

238. Pramono C. Surgical technique for achieving implant parallelism and measurement of the discrepancy in panoramic radiograph. J Oral Maxillofac Surg 2006; 64(5):799-803.

239. Proceedings of the 1996 World Workshop in Periodontics. Consensus report: Implant therapy II. Ann Periodontol 1996;1:816-20.

240. Rams TE, et al. The subgingival microflora associated with human dental implants. J Prosthet Dent 1984;5: 529-39.

241. Ravnholt G, Jensen J. Corrosion investigation of two material for implant. Superconstructions coupled to a titanium implant. Scand J Dent Res 1991;99:181-6.

242. Ravnholt G. Corrosion current, pH rise around titanium implants coupled to dental alloys. Scand J Dent Res 1998;96:466-72.

243. Reclaru L, Meyer JM. Study of corrosion between a titanium implant and dental Alloys. J Dent 1994;22: 159-68.

244. Rees TD. Periodontal management of the patient with diabetes mellitus. Periodontol 2000;23:63-72.

245. Reider C. A survey of natural tooth abutment intrusion with implant connected fixed partial dentures. IJ Periodont Restor Dent 1983;13:334-47.

246. Reiser GM, Nevins M. The implant periapical lesion: Etiology, prevention and treatment. Compend Contin Edu Dent 1995;16:768, 770, 772, Passim.

247. Report of the Expert Committee on the Diagnosis and Classification of Diabetes Mellitus. Diabetes Care 1997;20:1183-97.

248. Rhodus NL, Bloomquist C, Liljemark W, Bereuter J. Prevalence, density, and manifestations of oral *Candida albicans* in patients with Sjögren's syndrome. J Otolaryngol 1997;26:300-5.

249. Rhodus NL, Johnson DK. The prevalence of oral manifestations of systemic lupus erythematosus. Quintessence Int 1990;21:461-5.

250. Richard KK, George A Zarb, Adriamne Schmitt. Longitudinal peri-implant clinical responses in anterior mandibles of female patients: A preliminary report. J Prosthet Dent 1999;81:689-95.

251. Richey TK, Bennion SD. Etiologies of the sicca syndrome: Primary systemic amyloidosis and others. Int J Dermatol 1996;35:553-7.

252. Rissolo AR, Bennett J. Bone grafting and its essential role in implant dentistry. Dent Clin North Am 1998;42:91-116.

253. Robert Joffin, et al. Immediate loading of implants JP 2000;71:833-8.

254. Robert L Simon. Single implant supported molar and premolar crown - A 10-year retrospective clinical report. J Prosthet Dent 2003;90:517-21.

255. Roberts WE, Simmons KE, Garetto LP, DeCastro RA. Bone physiology and metabolism in dental implantology: risk factors for osteoporosis and other metabolic bone diseases. Implant Dent 1992;1:11-21.

256. Roberts WE, Smith RK, Zibermann Y, Mozsary PG, Smith RS. Osseous adaptation to continuous loading of rigid endosseous implants. Am J Orthod 1984;86:95-111.

257. Ryberg A. Mechanisms of chromium toxicity in mitochondria, Chem Biol Interact 1990;75:141-51.

258. Sack KE, Whitcher JP, Carterton NL, Greenspan JS, Daniels TE. Sarcoidosis mimicking Sjögren's syndrome: Histopathologic observations. J Clin Rheumatol 1998;4:13-6.

259. Sato N. Toward a more fundamental understanding of corrosion processes. Corrosion 1989;45:354-68.

260. SB Block Implants in dentistry edition 1997;62.

261. Sbordone L, Barone A, Ramaglia L, Ciaglia RN, Iacono VJ. Antimicrobial susceptibility of periodontopathic bacteria associated with failing implants. J Periodontol 1995;66:69-74.

262. Scarano A, Piattelli M, Vrespa G, Caputi S, Piatelli A. Bacterial adhesion on titanium nitride-coated and uncoated implants: An *in vivo* study. J Oral Implantol 2003;29(2):80-5.

263. Schein OD, Hochberg MC, Munoz B, Tielsch JM, Bandeen-Roche K, Provost T, et al. Dry eye and dry mouth in the elderly: A population-based assessment. Arch Intern Med 1999;159:1359-63.

264. Schliephake H, Charnweber D, Dard M, Robetalar S, Sewing A, Huttmann C. Biological performance of biomimetic calcium phosphate coating of titanium implants in the dog mandible. J Biomed Mater Res 2003;64A(2):225-34.

265. Schlosberg M, Movsowitz C, Epstein S, Ismail F, Fallon MD, Thomas S. The effect of cyclosporin: A administration and its withdrawal on bone mineral metabolism in the rat. Endocrinology 1989;124:2179-84.

266. Schnitman PA, Shulman LB: Dental implants, benefits and risks, proceedings of NIH Harvard Consensus Conference. 1978.

267. Shernoff AF, Colwell JA, Bingham SF. Implants for type II diabetic patients: Interim report. VA Implants in Diabetes Study Group. Implant Dent 1994;3:183-5.

268. Shetty V, Bertalami CN. The physiology of wound healing in Peterson LJ. Principles of oral and max surgery. Philadelphia, JB Lippincott, 1992;3-18.

269. Ship JA, Pillemer SR, Baum BJ. Xerostomia and the geriatric patient. J Am Geriatr Soc 2002;50:535-43.

270. Shulman LB. Dental implantation and transplantation. Laskin D oral and max surgery. Vol 2, Sl Louis, CV Mosby 1985;132, 133, 136.

271. Siegel MB, Potsic WP. Ectodermal dysplasia: The otolaryngologic manifestations and management. Int J Pediatr Otorhinolaryngol 1990;19:265-71.

272. Silverstein L, Garg A, Callan D, Shatz P. The key to success: Maintaining the long-term health of implants. Dent Today 1998;17:104, 106, 108-11.

273. Silverstein LH, Kurtzman GM. Oral hygiene and maintenance of dental implants. Dent Today 2006;25 (3):70-5 Quiz 75.

274. Skalak R. Biomedical considerations of osseointegrated prostheses. J Prosthet Dent 1983;49:483-8.

275. Smith and Zarb GA. Criteria for success of osseo-integrated endosseous implants. J Prosthet Dent 1989;62(6):567-72.

276. Smith RA, Berger R, Dodson TB. Risk factors associated with dental implants in healthy and medically compromised patients. Int J Oral Maxillofac Implants 1992;7:367-72.

277. Smith RA, Vargervik K, Kearns G, Bosch C, Koumjian J. Placement of an endosseous implant in a growing child with ectodermal dysplasia. Oral Surg Oral Med Oral Pathol 1993;75:669-73.

278. Snow ET, Xu L. Chromium (III) bound to DNA templates promotes increased plumerase processivity and decreased fidelity during replication vitro, Biochemistry 1991;30:238-45.

279. Soto-Rojas AE, Villa AR, Sifuentes-Osornio J, Alarcon-Segovia D, Kraus A. Oral candidiasis and Sjögren's syndrome. J Rheumatol 1998;25:911-5.

280. Spiekermann H, Jansen VK, Richter EJ. A 10-year follow-up study of IMZ and TPS implants in the edentulous mandible using bar-retained overdentures. Int J Oral Maxillofac Implants 1995;10:231-43.

281. Sreebny LM, Schwartz SS. A reference guide to drugs and dry mouth. 2nd edition. Gerodontology 1997;14:33-47.

282. Stearns DM, Courtne KD, Giangrande PH, Phieffer LS, Wetterhahn KE. Chromium (VI) reduction by ascorbate: role of reactive intermediates in DNA damage *in vitro*. Environ Health Persp 1994;102:21-5.

283. Stefano, et al. How different titanium surfaces affect osteoblast response. Journal of Periodontology 2004;75:273-82.

284. Steflik DE, Koth DC, Mc Kinney RV: Human Clinical trials with single crystal sapphire endosteal implant. J Oral Implant 1986;13:39-53.

285. Steiner M, Ramp WK. Endosseous dental implants and the glucocorticoid-dependent patient. J Oral Implantol 1990;16:211-7.

286. Steven E Haas. Implant supported, long-span fixed partial denture for a scleroderma patient: A clinical report. J Prosthet Dent 2002;87:136-9.

287. Steven J Sadowsky. Mandibular implant-retained overdentures: A literature review. J Prosthet Dent 2001;86:468-73.

288. Strock AE. Experimental work on dental implantation in the alveolus. Am J Orthod Oral Surg 1939;25:5, cited by Carl E Misch.

289. Sutow EJ, Jones DW, Milne EL. In Nitro Crevice Corrosion behavior of implant materials. J Dent Res 1985;64(5):842-7.

290. Takeshita F, Murai K, Iyama S, Ayukawa Y, Suetsugu T. Uncontrolled diabetes hinders bone formation around titanium implants in rat tibiae. A light and fluorescence microscopy, and image processing study. J Periodontol 1998;69:314-20.

291. Takuo Kuboki, Soichiro Okamoto, Hidenori Suzuki, Manabu Kanyama, Hikaru Arakawa, Wataru Sonoyama and Atsuski Yamashita. Quality of life assessment of bone-anchored fixed partial denture patients with unilateral mandibular distal extension edentulism. J Prosthet Dent 1999;82:182-7.

292. Tarlow, et al. Effect of adult growth on position of implant in anterior part of maxilla. JPD 2004;92: 213-5.

293. Tarnow DP, Emtiaz S, Classi A. Immediate loading of threaded implants at stage one surgery in edentulous arches: Ten consecutive case reports with 1-5 year data. Int J Oral Maxillofac Implants 1997;12:319-24.

294. Tarnow, et al. The effect of interimplant distance on the height of interimplant bone crest. JP 2000;71: 546-9.

295. Tatum OH. Osseous grafts in intraoral sites. J Oral Implantol 1996;22:51-2.

296. Tatum OH. the Omni Implant System, Birmingham, Ala, May 1988, Alabama Implant Congress.

297. Teerlinck J, Quirynen M, Darius MS, et al. Periotest, an objective clinical diagnosis of bone apposition towards implants. Int J Oral Maxillofac Impl 1991; 6(1): 55-61.

298. Ten Bruggenkate C, Vander Kwast WAM, Oosterbeek HS. Success criteria in oral implantology: A review of literature. Int J Oral Implant 1990;7:45-53.

299. Tinanoff N, Tanzer JM, Kornman KS, Maderazo EG. Treatment of the periodontal component of Papillon-Lefèvre syndrome. J Clin Periodontol 1986;13:6-10.

300. Tong-Mei Wang, et al. Intrusion and reversal of a natural tooth bounded by 2 implant supported prosthesis. JPD 2004;92:418-22.

301. Tortamano P, Orii TC, Yamanochi J, Nakamae AE, Guarnieri Tde C. Outcomes of fixed prostheses supported

by immediately loaded endosseous implants. Int J Oral Maxillofac Implants 2006;21(1):63-70.

302. Trakas T, Michalakis K, Kang K, Hirayama H. Attachment systems for implant retained overdentures: A literature review. Implant Dent 2006;15(1):24-34.

303. Triplett, et al. Endosseous cylindrical implants in severely atrophic mandibles. IJ Oral and Max surgery 1991;6:264-9.

304. Tseng CC. Periodontal status of patients with Sjögren's syndrome: A cross-sectional study. J Formos Med Assoc 1991;90:109-11.

305. Tseng CC, Wolff LF, Rhodus N, Aeppli DM. The periodontal status of patients with Sjögren's syndrome. J Clin Periodontol 1990;17:329-30.

306. Ullbro C, Crossner CG, Lundgren T, Stalblad PA, Renvert S. Osseointegrated implants in a patient with Papillon-Lefèvre syndrome. A 4 1/2-year follow-up. J Clin Periodontol 2000;27:951-4.

307. van der Reijden WA, Vissink A, Veerman EC, Amerongen AV. Treatment of oral dryness related complaints (xerostomia) in Sjögren's syndrome. Ann Rheum Dis 1999;58:465-74.

308. Venugopalan R, Linda C. Lucas Evaluation of restorative and implant alloys galvanically coupled to titanium. Dent Mater 1998;14:165-72.

309. von Wowern N, Klausen B, Kollerup G. Osteoporosis: A risk factor in periodontal disease. J Periodontol 1994;65:1134-8.

310. Wakley GK, Baylink DJ. Implants: Systemic influences. CDA J 1987;15:76-85.

311. Weber HP, Fiorellini JP, Buser DA. Hard-tissue augmentation for the placement of anterior dental implants. Compend Contin Educ Dent 1997;18:779-784,786-788,790-791.

312. Wetterhahn KE, Demple B, Kulesz Martin M, Copeland ES Carcinogenesis: A chemical pathology study section workshop, Workshop Report from the Division of Research Grants, National Institutes of Health. Cancer Res 1992;52:4058-63.

313. Wilson RM, Reeves WG. Neutrophil phagocytosis and killing in insulin-dependent diabetes. Clin Exp Immunol 1986;63:478-84.

314. Wood RE, Lee P. Analysis of the oral manifestations of systemic sclerosis (scleroderma). Oral Surg Oral Med Oral Pathol Oral Radiol Endod 1988;65:172-8.

315. World Health Organization. Assessment of fracture risk and its application to screening for post-menopausal osteoporosis: Report of a WHO study group. World Health Organ Tech Rep Ser 1994;843:1-129.

316. Yokoyama K, Ichikawa T, Murakami H, Miyamoto Y, Asaoka K. Fracture mechanisms of retrieved titanium screw thread in dental implant. Biomaterials 2002;23: 2459-65.

317. Young Hwan JO, Peter K Habo and Sumiya Hobo. Freestanding and multiunit immediate loading of the expandable implant: An upto 40 month prospective survival study. J Prosthet Dent 2001;85:148-55.

318. Yue S, Pilliar RM, Weatherly GC. The fatigue strength of porous coated Ti-6Al-4V implant alloy. J Biomed Mat Res 1984;18:1043-58.

319. Zarb, et al. Osseointegrated dental implants: Preliminary report on a replication study. JPD 1983;50:271-76.

320. Zarb GA, Schmitt A. The longitudinal clinical effectiveness of osseointegrated dental implants. The Toronto study. Part III: Problems and complications encountered. J Prosthet Dent 1990;64:185-94.

321. Zarb GA, Schmitt A. The longitudinal clinical effectiveness of osseointegrated dental implants. The Toronto study. Part I: Surgical results. J Prosthet Dent 1990;63:451-7.

322. Zarb GA, Schmitt A. The longitudinal clinical effectiveness of osseointegrated dental implants in posterior partially edentulous patients. Int J Prosthodont 1993;6:189-96.

Index